FAMILY CARERS AND CARING

T0267126

Family Carers and Caring: What It's All About
makes a major contribution to the current debate
about the future of social care in the UK and most
importantly offers the basis for a new and evidenced
narrative about how we identify, recognise and value
the family carers who form the bedrock of our
somewhat tired welfare state. Social care promised by
Boris Johnson on the steps of 10 Downing Street was
a historic moment to reconfigure our care system and
thereby to formally recognise, support but not
exploit the contributions of family cares. Delivery
was delayed, but that delay creates opportunity and
Family Carers and Caring offers the perfect brief for
reforms to come, acknowledging and evidencing the
critical role that family carers will play within a
redesigned care system.

Family carers, unpaid, often over-burdened and
poorly understood, underpin both the UK health and
the social care systems. The value of their care is
estimated at £193 billion a year, but there is growing
evidence of multiple health and financial inequalities
as carers care for longer and many struggle to
balance complex care at home with employment and
wider family responsibilities. Family care of necessity
has become a 21st-century issue for local and
national government. 1 in every 5 of NHS staff now
have family caring responsibilities. The UK
workforce needs to reverse the early retirement of so
many workers in middle age, many of whom have
acquired new caring responsibilities. We are seeing

*the rise of young carers whose own education and
career prospects are at risk because they are neither
recognised nor supported sufficiently. Additionally,
and importantly, the NHS is also reconfiguring the
role of hospitals and transferring health care and
recovery back into family homes.*

*The UK, of course, like its international counterparts,
has seen multiple strategies and new legislation over
the past two decades, intended to rebrand social care;
to integrate health and care and to personalise
support to meet individual needs. But family carers
have not achieved the 'parity of esteem' envisaged by
the Care Act and post-COVID financial challenges
mean that fewer carers are now receiving support. An
estimated 500,000 people await assessments or the
delivery of agreed packages of support from their
local authorities and families are still selling family
homes to pay for care. But even allowing for the very
real financial pressures on all public services, we can
do better and* **Family Carers and Caring** *offers
strategic analysis; creative forward thinking and a
new understanding of what 21st-century care and
support could look like.*

*As the authors note in the introduction to Chapter 2
of their book, the profile of the population of family
carers in the UK is dynamic, diverse and constantly
shifting. We are beginning to see the 'big
conversations' which have already taken place in a
number of our European neighbours around how we
define and therefore how we deliver social care and
support and the role of family carers in a changing
society. The House of Lords Adult Social Care
Committee recently entitled a report on the state of*

UK social care as 'A Gloriously Ordinary Life' *in recognition of powerful stories from family carers and those they support who wanted to reimagine care to actively support* 'ordinary lives' *and 21st-century preferences and ambitions. As a long-term personal carer myself, I can only hope that this book is read, discussed and shared across local and national government, the NHS and of course the UK's rich constellation of community organisations as we work together to define an* 'ordinary life' *for the extraordinary people who are family carers and how we can progressively and strategically work together to achieve it.*

Dame Philippa Russell DBE, Vice-President,
Carers UK

This excellent book presents a wide-ranging, informative and accessible discussion of what family care and carers are 'all about', *with conceptual and theoretical material illustrated by case studies. Drawing on their extensive knowledge of the subject, Milne and Larkin argue for change in the place of family care within social care systems. This book will be a valuable resource for a range of students and researchers in social work, social policy and related subjects.*

Professor Liz Lloyd, Senior Research Fellow,
School for Policy Studies, University of Bristol

FAMILY CARERS AND CARING

What It's All About

BY

ALISOUN MILNE

University of Kent, UK

And

MARY LARKIN

The Open University, UK

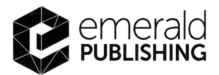

United Kingdom – North America – Japan – India
Malaysia – China

Emerald Publishing Limited
Howard House, Wagon Lane, Bingley BD16 1WA, UK

First edition 2023

Reprints and permissions service
Contact: www.copyright.com

British Library Cataloguing in Publication Data
A catalogue record for this book is available from the British Library

ISBN: 978-1-80043-349-6 (Print)
ISBN: 978-1-80043-346-5 (Online)
ISBN: 978-1-80043-348-9 (Epub)

INVESTOR IN PEOPLE

Alisoun dedicates the book to her husband Simon,
Mary dedicates the book to her eldest granddaughter Alice.
We would also both like to dedicate the book to those who do caring now and will become carers in the future.

CONTENTS

LIST OF FIGURES AND TABLES

Chapter 2

ABOUT THE AUTHORS

Alisoun Milne is Professor Emerita of Social Gerontology and Social Work at the University of Kent, UK. She has been involved in work on family caring for over twenty years; this included being a member of the independent advisory committee, the Standing Commission on Carers. Alisoun has written widely on care and caring issues and is embedded in national and international care-related research and practice networks. Up until 2021, Alisoun contributed to undergraduate and postgraduate social work programmes that included teaching on family care and carers.

https://www.kent.ac.uk/social-policy-sociology-social-research/people/1950/milne-alisoun-j

@alisounjm

Mary Larkin is Professor of Care, Carers and Caring at the Open University, UK. She has extensive experience of carer research and working with carers and carers organisations. Not only does she publish widely but her expertise in family caring has led to her membership of national and international bodies, committees and commissions. Mary's many years of teaching in higher education has included the development of courses about, and for, carers. Within the Open University she has spearheaded strategies to support students and staff who are carers.

https://www.open.ac.uk/people/mml5

1

INTRODUCTION

Family care is a prominent and universally challenging twenty-first century issue. At least 60% of UK adults will become a family carer at some point in their lives (Carers UK, 2019a; Organisation for Economic Co-operation & Development, 2021). Although it is now part of everyday discourse, the term 'carer' has been variously defined over time accommodating changes in the population as well as shifting understandings of issues such as age, culture, gender and what constitutes a 'family' (Larkin & Milne, 2014). This is reflected in its evolution from the focus solely on 'single women caring for elderly parents' to the contemporaneous widely accepted definition, that a carer is:

> *Anyone who cares, unpaid, for a friend or family member who due to illness, disability, a mental health problem or an addiction cannot cope without their support.*
> (Carers Trust: https://carers.org/about-caring/about-caring)

As this book will demonstrate, the concept remains contested. For many of those who actually 'do caring' the word carer has limited meaning; indeed, as many as half of carers do not own the term (Bowlby et al., 2010). Whilst acknowledging these tensions, the above definition is the one we have adopted for this book. The rationale for this decision is three-fold. The exploration of any group of people requires (some) clarity of definition. The Carers Trust definition not only offers us this, but it also makes explicit a key conceptual dimension of family caring, namely that carers are unpaid. Paid carers will be referred to (mainly) as care workers or care staff to avoid confusion. Whilst some terrain is shared by carers and care workers, for example gender issues, definitional differentiation is essential in order for us to be confident about the academic and experiential territory we are exploring in our book.

A third issue relates to a distinction between caring that is normative or 'usual', for example looking after a healthy child, and caring for a person with specific support needs because of illness or disability. Parents who are caring for a chronically ill or disabled child would usually be defined as 'carers', whereas parents with dependent children who do not have a long-term health condition or disability would not. The boundary between 'the family' and a 'family carer' is a fourth issue. We acknowledge that support and care by families take a number of forms and that family relationships intersect with caring ones. The focus of our book is on 'carers' and 'caring'; the wider impact of ill health and/or disability on relationships and families is addressed but not in any depth (Price & Walker, 2015).

The combination of cultural variation, contestation and definitional inconsistency means that the shape and profile of who is – and who is not – regarded as 'a carer' is dynamic and complex. Nonetheless, that the number of carers in the UK – and across the world – is increasing and is predicted to continue to increase is widely accepted. In 2021, it was estimated that there were 10.6 million carers in the UK and at least 647 million carers worldwide. 4.3 million people become carers every year in the UK; there are 12,000 'new' carers each day (Carers UK, 2022a). In 2001, 2% of the UK population were carers; by 2011 this figure had risen to 12%, and by 2019 it was 15%. Predictions pre-COVID-19 (COVID) suggested that by 2037 the number of carers in the UK will have increased to over 11 million (Brimblecombe et al., 2018a; Larkin & Milne, 2014). COVID led to a dramatic rise from 15% to 26%, i.e. 13.6 million people; an *additional* 4.5 million people started caring during the pandemic (Carers UK, 2020c). It is not known how many of these 'new' carers will become carers in the longer term, but it seems very likely a significant proportion will, increasing numbers still further.

There are a range of intersecting factors which have contributed to the increased demand for family care. The ageing profile of the UK – and worldwide – population is a key driver. There has also been a reduced use of institutional care; improvements in the lifespan of children and adults with lifelong disabilities; a continuing demographic shift to smaller more dispersed families; and cuts to support services for the carer *and* the cared-for person. The relatives that carers support now tend to be older and/or are much more dependent than they were 20 years ago; care tasks are also more demanding, time consuming and complex (Larkin et al., 2019). The policy context in which these socio-demographic changes have occurred is an additional key influence. Over the last 30 years social care policies have been underpinned by an assumption that people with dependency needs are best cared for by their relatives in the community and that reliance on public services is to be avoided except in the most extreme of circumstances. This is an issue to which we return in Chapter 4.

The carer population is not only changing in size but also in nature. It is estimated, for example, that the numbers of people taking on a caring role each year (pandemics excluded) is very similar to the number whose caring responsibilities come to an end. More carers are also undertaking serial caring roles; an increasing number are caring for an elderly parent, for example, and then later on in their life course, are caring for their spouse (Carers UK, 2021a).

In terms of who carers support, the most frequently identified conditions – in descending order of likelihood – are age-related health problems such as frailty and dementia; mental illness; people at the end of life and cancer (Larkin et al., 2019). Most carers support just one person (83%), although 14% care for two people and 3% are caring for three people or more (Carers UK, 2019a). This issue is explored in Chapter 2.

Caring roles and tasks range from the relatively moderate to the very intensive. Tasks include shopping, preparing meals, collecting medication, cleaning, doing the laundry, taking someone to medical appointments, administering medication, offering personal care (such as bathing and dressing), physical help (such as getting in and out of bed), social and emotional support, helping with financial matters and/or benefits, keeping an eye on the person, taking them out and organising formal services and/or professional care (Carers UK, 2019a; Larkin & Milne, 2014; Petrie & Kirkup, 2018). What carers do with, and for, the cared-for person varies depending on their level of need, their condition, what other kinds of support they receive (from other relatives or formal care services) and the nature of the care relationship.

The number of tasks and amount of care carers provide also varies; as might be expected, it reflects the nature and intensity of the care tasks. A carer might provide a few hours of care a week – shopping, collecting medication and taking someone to medical appointments – or may care 24/7. Those providing more intensive care such as personal and physical care tend to provide more hours of care per week (Carers UK, 2019a). More intensive carers tend to live with the person they support i.e. they are co-resident. Research from 2019 shows that on average carers in the UK provide 19.5 hours of care per week; just under half (48%) provide care for 20 or more hours; and a fifth (21%) care for more than 50 hours per week. Some carers care for many years; recent evidence suggests that over two-thirds of carers (65%) had been carers for over 5 years whilst almost a quarter (23.5%) had been caring for 20 years or more (NHS Digital, 2019).

In most middle- and high-income countries care of those with dependency needs would be unsustainable without the provision of family care. It represents 9% of global GDP (International Alliance of Carer Organisations, 2021). In the UK the economic value[1] of family care has been estimated to be £193 billion per year, outstripping the total cost of the National Health Service (NHS) (Carers UK, 2020a). In 2017 it was estimated that 149 million hours of care a week were being provided by family carers in the UK. At least an extra 4 million full-time care workers would be required if family carers ceased providing care tomorrow (Petrie & Kirkup, 2018).

WHY WRITE THIS BOOK?

Our intention in writing this book is to bring key dimensions of the carers discourse together – for the first time – into a single critical narrative presented in an accessible and yet academically informed way. Whilst there is a plethora of material on care and carers, it tends to be disparate, fragmented and located in a number of disciplinary spheres:

---

1 This is the cost of replacement care provided by unpaid carers based on an official estimate of the actual cost per hour of providing home care to an adult.

academic research, policy and service related material, carer
generated evidence, theoretical analysis, public health, social
care and social work, and work relating to rights, social justice
and inequalities.

Our aim is to help readers make sense of the complexities
of carers and caring and offer a 'way through' the carer
terrain. Given carers' contemporary and global significance
and the fact that family care is of growing public and policy
concern, the book is both timely and relevant to a wide target
population.

Carers are uniquely situated on the intersection of population ageing, social policy, the family, gender issues and the
role of the welfare state. Carers are both a public and a policy
issue and a private family matter (Phillips, 2007). They are the
focus of academic analysis and research and are of increasing
concern to services and care practice. Carers are enmeshed
with the concepts of care and caring, both conceptually and in
the language of the everyday. The very nature of care itself is
under scrutiny; questions about the boundary between the
informal sector and formal services, how far care is a 'task',
how far a 'duty' and how far 'a dimension' of all human
relationships infuses literature in both the academic and
non-academic spheres (Barnes, 2012).

How carers and caring are conceptualised is an important
issue as it shapes the nature and direction of policy. In turn,
policy shapes how care is arranged and organised and the role
of support services. In a context of welfare constraint, the
primacy of neo-liberal principles, and a strong emphasis on
'evidence of effectiveness' of services, carers tend to be conceptualised as unpaid members of the care workforce. Some
commentators – and carers – would say that carers are
exploited, expected to do the work of paid carers on an
unpaid and unsupported basis and there is well-documented
evidence about the negative implications of long-term

intensive caring for the physical and mental health of carers, their income and quality of life (Larkin et al., 2019: see Chapter 3).

The book's content and tone is informed by the lens of social and health related inequalities, offering a conceptual analysis that both extends understanding and challenges existing thinking in relationship to care and caring (Barnes, 2006; Larkin, 2011; Milne, 2020). It also makes visible issues of social justice. If we are to protect the well-being and rights of the growing number of carers and engage meaningfully with developing models of sustainable care for people with support needs, reframing 'carers issues' is an essential pre-requisite. Caring is explicitly a political issue as well as a personal, family and societal one.

Our book is made up of 7 chapters, including this one. Chapter 2 outlines the *Profile of Family Caring in the UK: Patterns and Trends*; the key dimensions of 'what we know' about carers (mainly) in the UK and what they do. Chapter 3 reviews the *Impact and Consequences of Caring on Carers*, including the range of negative emotional, financial and physical consequences linked to caring and also benefits associated with caring. Chapter 4 – *Supporting Carers* – outlines care-related policy and what is known about the role and effectiveness of services for carers. *Conceptualising and Understanding Care and Caring* is the focus of Chapter 5; it explores two key blocks of material, conceptual lenses on care and caring, and understanding the nature of care and caring. Chapter 6 – *Social Justice, Social Citizenship and Rights for Carers* – reviews the intersection between carers, social justice and rights and ways that these inform a fairer more egalitarian model of care and support for carers. In Chapter 7 – *Final Reflections: Looking Forward* – we offer a brief overview of the book's contribution to the public understanding of care, caring and carers and offer the reader some key 'takeaway' messages. Particular attention is paid to caring and inequalities. Whilst the book's chapters build on one another, they can stand alone; links between issues and chapters are made where useful. As COVID is a global issue of some significance, we have woven material relating to its implications for carers where relevant. We offer a number of case examples; for reasons of brevity we have been obliged to be mindfully selective.

We intend to achieve a balance between breadth and depth in the book. Whilst we identify different caring challenges and populations of carers, there are some groups we have not had room to include, e.g. carers of those with HIV/AIDS. We have said little about the role of friends or communities, not because we do not consider them to be important but because it is relatives who provide the majority of unpaid care. Our focus is primarily adult carers supporting another adult although we do refer to young (aged under 18 years) carers and parent carers of disabled children. As those carers who do more intensive levels and types of care are the most challenged, we pay particular attention to them. We also discuss policy and the law, but we are not addressing specific legal issues here; that is the role of more specialised texts. Whilst we acknowledge that care and caring are global issues, space does not permit country-specific analysis beyond the jurisdictions of the UK. With theories too we have inevitably engaged with those that have had the greatest influence on carer-related discourse, research and on contemporary understanding of care and caring.

2

PROFILE OF FAMILY CARING IN THE UK: PATTERNS AND TRENDS

INTRODUCTION

This chapter captures and explores the profile of family caring in the UK. The population(s) of carers is dynamic and shifting and intersects with a number of key dimensions of the UK's wider socio-demographic profile, for example the growing number of older people. Following a critical reflection on the dimensions and nature of data about carers, we will explore patterning, inequalities, trends and changes in the groups of people carers care for, carers' motivation for caring, the intensity of care provided and the profiles of a number of different sub-populations of carers. The chapter ends with an analysis of the key challenges facing UK society in relation to family caring.

CARER NUMBERS

Chapter 1 highlighted the growth in the number of carers in the UK and the dramatic rise since the pandemic began in early 2020: from 15% to 26% of the adult population. This means that up to 13.6 million people – one in four adults – are

Table 2.1. Number of Carers: Before and After the Coronavirus Pandemic.

Nation	Caring Pre-COVID	Caring Since COVID	Increase
Wales	19% (487,000)	27% (683,000)	8% (196,000)
Northern Ireland	15% (212,000)	22% (310,000)	7% (98,000)
Scotland	16% (729,000)	25% (1.1 million)	9% (392,000)

Source: Based on data from Carers UK (2020a, 2020b).

providing unpaid care in the UK today. The percentages of those caring across the UK[1] pre-pandemic varied as do the increases subsequent to it (see Table 2.1). As can be seen, 19% of the Welsh adult population said they were providing care before the pandemic; this is higher than both Northern Ireland and Scotland where the figures were 15% and 16%, respectively. The increases in each of these nations since the pandemic are all relatively close – 8% in Wales, 7% in Northern Ireland and 9% in Scotland (Carers UK, 2020a, 2020b).

Most of the enumerative data about carers are from national or regional censuses and surveys conducted either by leading carers organisations or via national research conducted by well-established research units (Milne & Larkin, 2015). Although helpful, these sources can be challenged. For example, the nature of questions about caring varies as does the definition of the term 'carer'; thus there are comparability issues. This can be illustrated with reference to census data. In

---

1 Data about England were not included in the available data sources.

response to public and policy interest in carers, a question about 'unpaid care', intended to establish the total number of carers in the UK, was introduced in the 2001 National Census. Following consultation and pilot testing, revised questions were included in the 2011 census and repeated in the 2021 census (Office for National Statistics, 2020). A specific revision to the 2021 questions includes omission of the word 'unpaid' to avoid confusion with other activities such as care of a non-disabled child or volunteering. In 2011, a broader definition of carer was also introduced, i.e. 'anyone' instead of 'family members, friends, neighbours or others'. The question asked is in Box 2.1.

Despite the fact that questions about carers are now included in the Census, and other large-scale surveys, it is widely accepted that these data sources are likely to significantly underestimate the total number of carers. They tend not to capture those who adopt the role for a temporary period, such as carers of people who recover from an illness. Nor do they reflect carers who move in and out of a caring role, for example supporting a person who has an episodic mental illness, or carers whose caring role has a clear 'end point', such

---

Box 2.1

Census 2021 'Are You a Carer?' Question

Do you look after, or give any help or support to, anyone because they have any long-term physical or mental health conditions or illnesses, or problems related to old age?

Source: *Office for National Statistics (2023).*

as those caring for a relative with a terminal condition
(Argyle, 2016; Askey et al., 2009). There are concerns about
the accuracy of the Census data for 2021 as it was conducted
during a worldwide pandemic.

A linked point, and a very important one in terms of data
accuracy, is the fact that a lot of carers simply do not identify
as 'a carer'. For many of those who actually 'do caring', the
term carer has limited meaning (Carers UK, 2016). Indeed,
some commentators maintain that it is a bureaucratically
generated notion turning 'what is a normal human experience
into an unnecessarily complex phenomenon' (Molyneaux
et al., 2011, p. 422). Most carers take years to recognise their
role (if they ever do). Research shows that over half of carers
(54%) take more than a year to do so, nearly a quarter (24%)
take over 5 years and nearly 1 in 10 (9%) take over 10 years.
Whilst this partly reflects the fact that carers tend to gradually
adopt the role of carer over time – rarely is there a single
moment when someone 'becomes' a carer – it is also reflective
of the conceptual status of 'carer'. Many spouses, in particular, would never be willing to call themselves a carer as it
undermines the very essence of marriage and the mutuality of
the relationship. This is an issue to which we return in later
chapters.

Despite the shortcomings of data on carers, as the discussions in the rest of this chapter will demonstrate, it does offer
useful insights into patterns of family caring in the UK.

WHO DO CARERS SUPPORT?

Only 1 in 10 carers (9%) care for a friend or neighbour; the
majority of carers care for a relative. The most recent data
show that two-fifths of carers (41%) care for their parents or

parents-in-law; over a quarter (26%) care for a spouse or partner; 8% care for a disabled child (under 18 years of age); 5% are looking after an adult son or daughter with disabilities; 4% are caring for a grandparent(s); and 7% care for 'another relative' such as a sibling, aunt or cousin (See Fig. 2.1). Over half (58%) of the cared-for population have a physical disability, one-fifth (20%) have a sensory impairment, 13% have a mental health problem and 10% have dementia (Department for Work and Pensions, 2020).

Familial care relationships are typically either dyadic – such as between co-habiting spouses or parent and child – or non-dyadic. Examples of non-dyadic relationships include those between daughters and sons in law caring for elderly parents/in law, and grandchildren caring for a grandparent. Dyadic carers are nearly always co-resident; non-dyadic carers tend to be extra-resident i.e. the carer and cared-for person live in separate homes.

'Family' and 'relationship' are central to understanding who carers support. Although family structures vary between cultures, social classes and generations, the term 'family' is

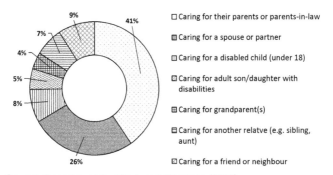

Source: Department for Work and Pensions (2020).

Fig. 2.1. Who Carers Support.

universally associated with notions of duty, obligation, attachment, responsibility and reciprocity. It remains a fundamental building block of care for those with dependency needs across the globe (Bowlby et al., 2010; Mason & Finch, 1993).

An example of how the concept of family changes over time is the shift – in the West at least – over the past few decades from the family as comprising a co-resident hetero-sexual married couple with (shared) children to encompassing a broad range of different relationships and models. These include, second or even third marriages with step-children, long-term non-legal partnerships, same-sex marriages/civil unions and lone parents. These changes may mean that caring relationships take a number of new and different forms in the future. For example, caring may be shared to a greater degree than is the case now between, step-children, half siblings and ex-partners (Greenwood & Smith, 2019). The 'reconstituted' family will be a particular influence on patterns of caring.

REASONS FOR THE NEED FOR CARE

Further analysis of data about the cared-for population shows that a large percentage (70%) are parents/in law or spouses/partners who are aged over 65 years with age-related disabilities, e.g. sensory impairments, dementia and/or mobility issues or chronic physical and mental health conditions. Key health issues or conditions that require carer input amongst younger adults are: learning disabilities, mental health problems, a terminal illness (such as cancer), alcohol or drug dependency, and (increasingly) diabetes (Carers UK, 2019a; Public Health England, 2021).

That population ageing is a key driver behind the increased demand for family care was discussed in Chapter 1. This warrants more in-depth exploration in terms of changes in the profile of the cared-for population. In 2016, it was estimated that 11.8 million people – 18% of the population – were aged over 65 years. This is expected to increase to 19.8 million people, accounting for 26.2% of the population, by 2041. The increase in the proportion of those aged over 65 masks the even more rapid growth in those aged 80 years and over: a group often referred to as the 'older old'. The number of individuals in this age group is expected to double between 2016 and 2041 from 1.6 million to 3.3 million (Office for National Statistics, 2019; Petrie & Kirkup, 2018). Despite improvements in life expectancy and healthy life expectancy, as already indicated, the likelihood of being disabled and/or experiencing a range of chronic comorbid health conditions increases with age. Older people are more likely than younger people to have one or more long-term conditions. More than half (58%) of those aged over 60 have at least one long-term health condition, and a quarter (25%) have two or more; this is particularly the case for those aged over 80. There is a second trend to note. Although people are *generally* living longer, the number of years spent in poor health or with a disability is also extending. The proportion of our lives that we now can expect to live in poor health or with a disability has risen to just over a quarter (See Fig. 2.2: Centre for Ageing Better, 2021). Average life expectancy is now stalling and is even reducing amongst people whose lives are characterised by socio-economic disadvantage.

Overall, population ageing means that there are an increasing number of older people with dependency needs living in the community. Current predictions suggest that there will be a 113% increase in this number by 2051; needs are likely to be multiple and complex (Alzheimer's Society,

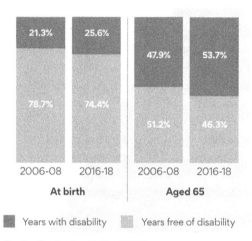

Source: Centre for Ageing Better (2021).

Fig. 2.2. Proportion of Life Spent with and without Disability at Birth and Age 65 (England).

2020; Public Health England, 2021). The implications for carers are twofold: more family members will be expected to provide care for their elderly relatives and caring demands will be greater. Carers will be supporting older people with co-morbidities, such as dementia *and* mobility problems, who require more, and more intensive, types of care.

A more hidden implication of the ageing population is the growth in the number of older carers; it is not just those who need care who are older, the profile of carers is ageing too. Over a third of all carers in the UK are aged over 65 and their numbers are rising (Larkin et al., 2020): this is explored in more detail below. Older carers may have their own health problems, often made worse by providing care. With spouse carers in particular, there is often a blurring of the distinction between 'carer' and 'cared-for person': they both need help from, and care for, the other. For example, one partner may be physically fit but has dementia and the other partner has cognitive capacity but is physically frail (Bowlby et al., 2010; Rapaport & Manthorpe, 2008). This is described as co-caring or mutual care.

That care demands are increasing is not just about the ageing population. As noted in Chapter 1, there is also improved longevity for children and younger adults with complex health-related needs and/or disabilities. This population(s) often need long-term care and support. As a consequence of advances in medical treatments and care, more babies born prematurely are surviving into adulthood; they are often vulnerable to experiencing multiple lifelong health conditions. A second issue is recent improvements in the life expectancy of children and adults with physical and learning disabilities, particularly those with learning disabilities (Larkin et al., 2019). For example, in 1983 the average lifespan of a person with Down syndrome was 25 years, whereas today it is approximately 60 years and is continuing to rise. Mortality for those with severe cerebral palsy has shifted from childhood to early adulthood; 40% of people with the condition are now likely to live to the age of 20 (Blair et al., 2019).

These socio-demographic trends, in combination with reduced use of long-term (institutional and hospital) care, a policy emphasis on the benefits of community-based care and reductions in spending on social care means that there is a *much* greater reliance on family carers to provide support to both younger and older adults with complex long-term needs (Brimblecombe et al., 2018a; Larkin & Milne, 2014; Malli et al., 2018). This expectation has profound implications for carers.

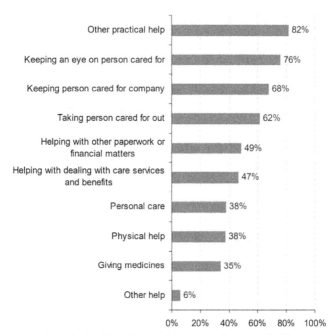

Source: The Health & Social Care Information Centre (2010).[2]

Fig. 2.3. Types of Help Provided for People Being Cared for.

CARE INTENSITY

The wide-ranging practical, physical and emotional activities and tasks that carers undertake were outlined in Chapter 1. Further details of these can be found in Fig. 2.3.

Care intensity is reflective of both the types of care tasks a carer does and the time taken to do them. These two factors intersect; the more complex a care task is, the more time it takes to complete, e.g. providing personal care (Carers UK, 2019b).

---

2 These are the most recent figures available.

Conversely, a simple care task such as picking up medication from the chemists is quickly and easily achieved. It is important to note that a carer who does personal care for a relative will also tend to do the less intensive care tasks as well (this is discussed further in Chapter 5). Care intensity is additive. It is usually enumerated by number of 'hours per week' (pw). This is an important barometer of the shifting nature of care. More people providing intensive care, i.e. more hours pw, reflects the more complex needs profile of those being cared for and the more demanding nature of care. That the number of carers caring round the clock (i.e. for 50 or more hours each week) increased by 25% between 2008 and 2018 (Carers UK, 2019b) is clear evidence of this changing pattern. The most recent figures (see Fig. 2.4) show that in 2018/9 14% of carers cared for over 50 hours per week (Department for Work and Pensions, 2020). It is clear that there are differences between female and male carers; this is an issue explored later in this chapter and in Chapter 3 too.

The proportion of carers providing 20 or more hours of care per week is gradually increasing too (Office for National Statistics, 2023). The figure rose from 24% to 28% between 2005 and 2015; it now accounts for nearly 50% of all carers. It

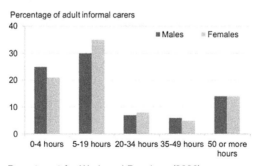

Source: Department for Work and Pensions (2020).

Fig. 2.4. Hours of Care Provided by Adult Family Carers per Week, by Gender, 2018/2019, United Kingdom.

is likely that the number of family carers providing intensive care will continue to increase for the foreseeable future. This reflects the nature of the care demands related to the conditions experienced by those being cared for as well as limited access to support, particularly social care services (discussed in Chapter 4) (Carers UK, 2019b; Petrie & Kirkup, 2018). During the pandemic, carers reported providing – on average – 10 *additional* hours of care per week as a consequence of: challenges related to using protective measures such as face masks, lack of external support from family and friends and very limited access to care and support services for the cared-for person (Carers UK, 2020a, 2020c; Cipolletta et al., 2021).

As most data on care intensity are collected via surveys, they only provide a snapshot at a single point in time. It does not tell us about care intensity across the whole trajectory of caring nor about how care demands change through time. Whilst for some carers, adopting the role may happen suddenly, such as in the case of a mother who gives birth to a disabled child or a husband whose wife has had a road traffic accident, research shows that for most carers' care intensity increases over time in response to their relative's (usually) deteriorating condition. Carers may begin with relatively undemanding tasks such as shopping or collecting medications and then, as the cared-for person becomes frailer and/or their needs become more complex (e.g. as with dementia), the carer increases their input accordingly.

Carers may eventually provide hands-on intensive care such as bathing, dressing and quasi-medical tasks (for example, monitoring intravenous medication or changing dressings) 24/7 (Larkin & Milne, 2014). As Bowlby et al. (2010) state, 'Caring can be viewed as a continuum along which family members move over time from reciprocal exchanges of help, to the provision of modest levels of assistance, and for some, ultimately to situations requiring intensive levels of care for a highly dependent person' (p. 43). The

latter stages of caring can mean that it becomes 'boundless. . ..
virtually limitless. . .. (often) characterised by spontaneous,
unexpected events or crisis which could occur at any time,
with demands being made during the night experienced as
particularly onerous' (Pickard & Glendinning, 2002, p. 148).
Evidence suggests that carers find caring for relatives with
dementia and/or multiple health problems especially challenging (Larkin et al., 2019). Research about care intensity
and the care journey interleaves with conceptual models of
care and theoretical issues relating to caring; these are discussed in Chapter 5.

Around half of carers support someone in the same
household (i.e. they are co-resident) and half support someone
in a separate household (i.e. they are extra resident). As noted
above, residency and whether a care relationship is dyadic or
not are linked; spouses and partners are, axiomatically,
co-resident as are most parent carers. Filial carers, i.e. sons/
daughters supporting a parent, are much more likely to be
extra resident. Location of care plays an important role in
relationship to care intensity. Co-resident carers are *much*
more likely than extra resident carers to provide intensive care
and perform more challenging care tasks, such as personal
care (54% co-resident compared with 22% for extra resident),
physical help (49% compared with 25%) and giving medication (50% compared with 18%). Although extra resident
carers tend to provide lower levels of intensive care, they often
have to travel to provide support. It is estimated that over a
quarter of extra resident carers live more than half an hour
away from their relative; this includes 6% who are obliged to
travel for over two hours to visit. These 'distance carers' tend
to be middle-aged sons or daughters/in law; they are more
likely to be combining caring with paid work and often with
the care of (older) children too (Carers UK, 2019b; Petrie &
Kirkup, 2018).

One potential consequence of increasing intensity of care for carers is the need to involve formal care services; this is something that tends to be delayed or avoided by the cared-for person and, often, by the carer too. This reluctance is driven by a number of intersecting factors: a belief that 'normality' can best be preserved through maintaining the person's independence; that if care is needed, it is the family's duty to provide it; and concerns about abuse or neglect by services. However, there is a tension between these drivers, and the huge weight of caring responsibilities growing numbers of carers are taking on for very ill or frail relatives some of whom require specialist care (Heath et al., 2018; Manthorpe et al., 2003). The policy emphasis on extending community-based living for all those with dependency needs has driven a 'shift in the locus of care' (McGarry, 2009, p. 83) from care homes and hospitals to the person's own home. Not only has this placed more demands on carers but, as a consequence of reduced input from nurses and other health-care staff, carers are now expected to do a set of tasks once done by trained health professionals (Bradley, 2015; Lilleheie et al., 2020). Increasingly carers are expected to monitor medication drivers (for example, for pain relief), ensure pills are taken on time and/or change dressings. There are ethical questions about whether it is right that untrained family carers do these tasks and whether they can do them safely too. There is a related question about the extent to which an overstretched care system expects – nee requires – this of carers. We return to this issue in Chapter 5.

An important contextual issue is reduced access to health and social care services. Over the last 10 years significant cuts have been made to welfare services for adults with dependency needs *and* their carers; this constitutes a 'double whammy' for carers. So-called austerity measures have resulted in the raising of eligibility criteria for accessing publicly funded social care to a very high level. This has, inevitably, placed additional pressure on carers despite legislative claims to the contrary (Malli et al., 2018) (also see Chapter 4). This pattern was amplified during the pandemic due to the partial or full closure of many health and social care services for users, requiring carers to 'pick up the care tab' to an even greater degree than hitherto. They also had to (often) manage alone as family and friends were unable to visit or offer help (Carers UK, 2020b, 2020c; Lafferty et al., 2022).

As a consequence of the shrinking availability of publicly funded care increasing numbers of people are obliged to purchase their own support from independent sector services, this group are called self-funders. Although there are no definitive numbers of self-funders, estimates suggest it is now in the region of 25% of all those in need of social care support. Finding and managing one's own care package can be challenging. Being a care 'consumer' is no guarantee of quality or efficiency and the additional costs of care can mean that people struggle to purchase sufficient care services to meet all of their needs. In these circumstances, carers often have to step in to make up any care shortfalls; they also (often) have to help their relative manage the whole process of self-funding. If a user and carer do not meet their local authority's eligibility criteria to receive support *and* have no money to fund their own care they are, simply, expected to manage. There is evidence that many carers feel 'coerced' into doing (even more) caring, giving up paid employment to provide care and/or topping up payments for care services from their own financial resources (Office for National Statistics, 2021; Tanner et al., 2022; Ward et al., 2020).

WHY CARERS CARE?

Despite their familial basis, it cannot be assumed that caring relationships are motivated by love, nor that they are entered into willingly; many carers feel obliged to care and that they have no choice in adopting the role. This is particularly the case for those who take on the care of an elderly parent (Larkin & Milne, 2014). Being reluctant to take on the caring role has been found to be associated with a number of (more) negative outcomes: poorer quality care, higher levels of abusive behaviour towards care recipients and more care arrangements breaking down (Greenwood & Smith, 2019). It may well be that more relatives will simply not be willing to take on the caring role in the future knowing that once entered into, it is almost impossible to give up, even when it is very damaging to the carer's own health and well-being. However, at present there is no evidence at all that families are withdrawing from caring. The vast majority of family members appear willing to care for a relative who becomes ill, especially in the early stages of that illness (Larkin et al., 2019). How care is understood as a 'family issue' and how care and caring are conceptualised is the focus of Chapter 5.

KEY DIMENSIONS OF THE CARER POPULATION

In this chapter we have explored the profile of the UK's carer population. Although we have been obliged to present the material in 'sections', we recognise that this is an imperfect process. Carers issues intersect and overlap in ways that defy boundaries.

This is further evidenced in the use of structural dimensions and categorisation by 'group' to disaggregate carers. Arguably, these partly reflect what policymakers and research funders want to know about, for example how to retain working carers in employment. Exploration of these two forms of disaggregation also shows us how the many faces of caring intersect with inequalities.

Structural dimensions commonly addressed within the care-related literature are gender, age, socio-economic status, race and sexuality (Ridley et al., 2010). These are explored below.

Gender

As Fig. 2.5 shows, there is a clear gender gradient in the carer population; approximately 60% of carers are women. There is also evidence that since 2010, whilst the overall proportion of caring done by women has increased by 11%, it has only increased by 3% for men. Gender also intersects with hours of care in that women provide on average 30% more hours of

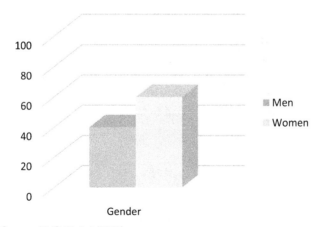

Source: NHS Digital (2019).

Fig. 2.5. Carers by Gender and Hours of Care per Week.

care a week than men. The increase in care intensity experienced by carers during the COVID pandemic referred to
above was far greater for women than men. In addition,
women are more likely than men to combine caring with
raising children. This gender imbalance exists across the
whole of the adult life course *except* in later life. For those
aged between 75 years and 84 years the gender split is 50:50;
in those aged over 85 years carers are more likely to be male
(59%) than female (41%) (Petrie & Kirkup, 2018; Seedat &
Rondon, 2021). The majority of this group of male carers are
spouses.

The gender imbalance in caring has been explored through
a number of academic lenses. Sociological explanations have
emphasised expectations relating to traditional gender roles,
i.e. that women are socialised to adopt the role of carer.
Theories of segregation of labour suggest that since women
are more likely to stay at home, it is 'natural' for them to
adopt the carer role and/or feel more obliged to give up paid
work to care (Sharma et al., 2016; Yeandle et al., 2017). The
gender rebalancing after the age of 75 is explained by the
pattern of spousal care in later life; as many, or more, husbands provide care for their wives as wives for their husbands.
This suggests something particular about the role of marriage,
especially long-term marriage, as a driver for providing care
amongst men (Larkin et al., 2020). The intersection of gender
and caring is further explored in Chapter 5.

Age

Although anyone of any age can become a carer, analysis of
the age distribution of carers shows that currently, around 2%
of carers are aged under 18 years, 3% are aged between 18
and 25 years, more than 50% are aged 40–64 years and 33%

are aged 65 years or over. Almost 30% of those who belong to the over 65's cohort are aged over 80 years. The peak age for providing care is 50–64 years; one in five people in this age group are carers (Age UK, 2019; Carers UK, 2019b; Department for Work and Pensions, 2020).

That population ageing means that a third of all carers in the UK are now aged 65+ and that their numbers are rising was referred to above. The overall profile of carers is ageing. The number of carers aged 65 and over is increasing more rapidly than the overall carer population, the greatest increase being amongst those aged 85+ years. This is termed the ageing of caring (Age UK, 2019; Carers UK, 2019b).

Socio-Economic Status

Evidence suggests an association between socio-economic factors and caring. Family care is more prevalent amongst those on lower incomes living in deprived areas compared with higher income groups living in wealthier areas (Bambra et al., 2020). This is due to a combination of factors. Life course exposure to health risks is greater amongst those who are socio-economically disadvantaged; this reflects the so-called social gradient in health (see Chapter 6). There is also a greater reliance on publicly funded care amongst those on lower incomes (Marmot et al., 2020). As already noted, public services have been significantly reduced in recent years. This has a disproportionate impact on poorer carers and the relatives they support. There are also differences between occupational groups in terms of intensity. Carers in higher occupational groups tend to provide fewer hours of care per week than those in the lower occupational groups as they are more likely to have the financial resources to self-fund

privately sourced services, such as home care (Hoff, 2015;
Public Health England, 2021).

Race

Whilst it is estimated that 10% of carers in the UK are from a
Black and Minority Ethnicity (BAME) background, we still
know relatively little about this population(s). This can be
partly attributed to the fact that rates of self-identification
tend to be lower amongst BAME carers; many consider
'carer' to be a 'culturally inappropriate' (Lloyd, 2006, p. 954)
term and antithetical to normal family relations (James,
2019). Nonetheless, there is evidence that BAME families are
more likely to provide care for older or disabled relatives than
white families. In addition, BAME carers are more likely to
care more intensively than other groups of carers and are
more reluctant to ask for help from services (Carers UK, 2011,
2019b).

Research into care and migration in the European Union
shows that families can be widely dispersed across different
countries. Many migrants (particularly those who are female)
feel under pressure, or wish to, move to another country in
order to provide or receive care at some point in their lives
(Larkin et al., 2019). The impact of Brexit on EU patterns of
family care are, as yet, unknown (Koffman et al., 2020).

Sexuality

It is estimated that 4% of carers are lesbian, gay, bisexual and
transgender (LGBTQ+). As with BAME and older carers,
reluctance to self-identify means that this figure is likely to be
much higher (Carers UK, 2019b). There is relatively little

literature on this group of carers. The evidence we do have highlights the extent to which heteronormative assumptions by health and social care professionals and services mean that many LGBTQ+ carers experience stigmatisation, their needs are often overlooked, they face difficulties in being accepted as 'next of kin' and they are often excluded from critical discussions and decisions relating to the cared-for person (Larkin et al., 2019; Willis et al., 2011).

The disaggregation of carers into groups is problematic as categorisations tend to suggest rigid distinctions between 'types' of carers or caring activities. These rarely exist. For instance, it is not uncommon for carers to straddle two or more groups (e.g. older carer/dementia carer), and there is considerable overlap in group characteristics. It is nevertheless useful for us to explore groups that are particularly prominent and/or who are growing in number. Although these groups are by no means comprehensive, they illustrate the complexity of the profile of 'who cares' and the breadth of the carer diaspora.

Working carers: not only has the carer population increased, but the proportion of working carers has also increased. Just over half (53%) of family carers are currently in paid work, which means that around one in nine workers in the UK has caring responsibilities. Two-thirds work full time and one-third part time (Carers UK, 2019a; Department for Work and Pensions, 2020). Fig. 2.6 (based on data from 2018/2019) provides information about the employment status and gender of those caring before the pandemic. 43% of female carers and 25% of male carers were working full time; in contrast, less than 10% of female but 23% of male carers were working part time. When these figures are broken down further they show that it is women working in professional and managerial roles that make up a growing proportion of the overall population of women who balance family care

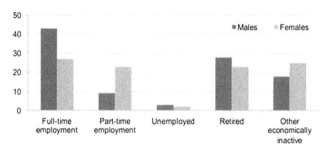

Source: Department for Work and Pensions (2020).

Fig. 2.6. Adult Carers Employment Status and Gender, 2018/2019.

with remaining in employment. This point intersects with that made above about carers in higher occupational groups providing fewer hours of care and paying for their own support services (self funding). Analyses of the age of working carers show that one in four older (50+) female workers, and one in eight older male workers, have caring responsibilities (Ní Léime et al., 2019; Petrie & Kirkup, 2018).

Sandwich carers: this group of carers is defined as those people who care for an older, sick or disabled relative at the same time as they are providing support for their own children and sometimes grandchildren too (Buckner & Yeandle, 2015; Do et al., 2014). They are a relatively new group of carers; their emergence can be attributed to the intersection of the growth in the number of older relatives with care needs – usually an elderly parent/in law – with a growth in the number of adult sons and daughters living with their parents, i.e. 25+ year olds. As both these trends continue, the number of sandwich carers is also likely to increase. In 2018 it was estimated that 3% of the UK population – equivalent to more than 1.3 million people – were sandwich carers. The peak age for sandwich caring is 40–44 years for women and 45–49 years for men. As might be expected, women are much more likely to be sandwich carers than men (Carers UK, 2019b). Recent empirical data in a range of European countries show that this gendered profile is shared; they reflect the common pattern of daughters/in law being expected to care for their parents/in law rather than sons. This risk is *not* reduced by active engagement in childcare and has been referred to as the 'sibship unequal distribution of care' (Luppi & Nazio, 2019, p. 779).

Young carers: a young carer is a child or young person under the age of 18 who looks after a relative who has a need for support. They may have a physical disability, a long-term illness, a mental health problem or drug/alcohol dependency. It is estimated that there are 800,000 young carers in the UK. However, many young carers remain hidden from view which means that this figure is likely to be an underestimate (Children's Society, 2020; Hounsell, 2013). Fig. 2.7 shows the different family members young carers support; most care for a parent or sibling. There is also evidence that older children are more likely than younger children to be taking care of their mother (58% of 16- to 17-year-old carers) whilst the youngest carers are more likely to be helping to care for a disabled or ill sibling (Cheesbrough et al., 2017; Children's Society, 2020).

The average age of a young carer is 12. However, for most young carers caring begins when they are young children; caring both continues, and increases in intensity, throughout their entire childhood, and sometimes beyond (Becker & Becker, 2009). Young carers consistently take on more responsibility than their peers for the management of their own lives and those of their relative. They undertake a wide spectrum of caring activities ranging from practical tasks (such as cooking, cleaning and paperwork) to helping a parent to bathe a disabled brother or sister, to being the sole

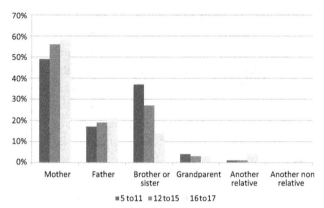

Source: Cheesbrough et al. (2017).

Fig. 2.7. Who Young Carers Care for by Age Group.

supporter for a lone parent with a severe mental health condition. It is estimated that one in four young carers (25%)
provide 'nursing care' (Cheesbrough et al., 2017). Although
the majority provide care for under 20 hours a week, thou-
sands provide higher levels of care, with over 10% providing
weekly care of 50 or more hours. COVID has significantly
increased young carers caring responsibilities. 58% reported
that they were spending an average of an additional 10 hours
a week on their caring role as a result of the pandemic
(Children's Society, 2020; Powell et al., 2020).

Despite only representing 2% of the total carer population,
young carers have attracted a great deal of policy and research
attention. The reasons for this appear to be two-fold. Young
carers can be profoundly disadvantaged by caring. Caring at a
young age can have life course implications for psychological
and physical health, friendships, and educational and occupational outcomes (see Chapter 3). There is additional evidence that the children most at risk of becoming young carers

are from disadvantaged backgrounds; they are more likely to live in low-income households and are over four times more likely to live in a household where no adults are in paid work. Young carers are also one and a half times more likely than their peers to have a special educational need or a disability. Furthermore, young carers in BAME communities – and there are proportionately more young carers in these communities (see Fig. 2.8) – are twice as likely not to speak English as their first language (James, 2019).

A second reason why young carers are the focus of policy concern is the widespread public unease about the extent to which children *should be* involved in caring (Aldridge, 2008; Hounsell, 2013). It intersects with issues of child protection, including 'harm' done to children by caring activities and whether these activities are 'appropriate' to the age and understanding of the child (Lloyd, 2023). It also shines a light on the state's responsibility for adults with health problems or a disability. After all, young carers are often substituting for

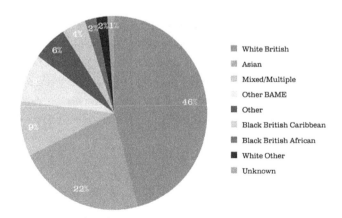

Source: James (2019).

Fig. 2.8. Ethnicity of Young Carers.

services the adult with care and support needs has a right to but the state has failed to provide.

Whilst it is entirely justified for us to explore the needs and profile of young carers, it is nonetheless noteworthy that research funders prioritise some groups of carers over others. This tendency produces an uneven, perhaps even unbalanced, evidence and knowledge base. We return to this issue later in the book.

Older carers: many older carers care for their spouses or partners. There are also other groups. For example, a quarter of all older carers are parents supporting an, often middle-aged, disabled son or daughter due to the increase in the longevity of adults with physical and/or learning disabilities (noted above). There is also a growing number of daughters aged 65 years or over caring for a *very* elderly parent.

Older carers usually have to cope with multiple complex needs and undertake intensive caring which routinely includes personal care, quasi-medical care and help with mobility issues (Petrie & Kirkup, 2018; Public Health England, 2021). Indeed, survey data show that older carers are more likely than other groups of carers to be providing intensive care and to care for many hours per week (Office for National Statistics, 2023). As Fig. 2.9 shows the hours of care pw increases as the carer ages, with carers aged 85 years and over providing the most intensive levels of care. In addition, older carers are often managing their own health and disability issues alongside caring (Larkin et al., 2020).

A particular feature of caring in later life is care of a spouse or partner. This typically takes place in the context of a long-term reciprocal relationship and beliefs about the 'care contract' that underpins marriage (or a similar relationship). As a consequence of the long-term and embedded nature of

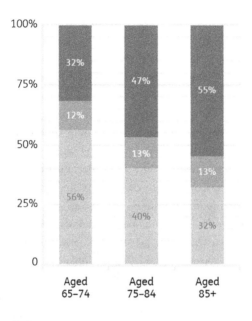

Provides **1–19 hrs** unpaid care a week

Provides **20–49 hrs** unpaid care a week

Provides **50 hrs or more** unpaid care a week

Source: White (2013).[3]

Fig. 2.9. Hours of Care Per Week Increases with Age.

their caring role, many older spouses do not identify as a carer (Hyden & Nilsson, 2015; Perkins, 2010; Pickard, 2010).

Dementia carers: it is older carers, particularly those aged 85 and over, who are most likely to be a carer for a spouse or a partner with dementia. It is estimated that there are currently over 700,000 dementia carers in the UK; at least 60% are

---

3 The 2021 Census had not, at the time of publication, provided more recent data.

women, primarily wives or daughters (Carers UK, 2021a; Wittenberg et al., 2019).

Studies show that caring for someone with dementia tends to be complex, demanding and intensive. This is partly a reflection of the nature of the condition itself and also because 80% of people living with dementia have at least one other condition. 36% of dementia carers are caring for more than 100 hours per week. They also tend to care over many years: around 30% of dementia carers care for over 5 years and a quarter care for more than 10 years. Coping with dementia-related symptoms, which often worsen as the condition progresses, is a particular challenge: these include dementia-related behavioural issues such as wandering and aggression, personality changes and incontinence (Alzheimers Society, 2020). It is estimated that there are currently around 900,000 people living with dementia in the UK, a figure that is projected to increase to 2 million by 2051. Given the likely increase (see Fig. 2.10), and the fact that care homes are increasingly reserved for those with very high levels of need, it is very likely that there will be a commensurate growth in the number of dementia carers (Larkin et al., 2020; Prince et al., 2014).

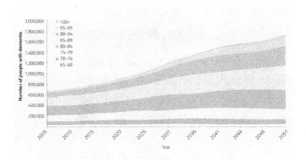

Source: Prince et al. (2014): Alzheimer's Society.

Fig. 2.10. Projected Increase in the Number of People with Dementia in the UK to 2051, by Age Group.

Dementia carers faced unprecedented challenges during the pandemic. People living with dementia experienced particularly severe symptoms from the virus *and* are also (generally) less able to understand, or remember, the rules relating to PPE and other protective measures. When a person with dementia does contract the virus, it often results in delirium, aggression and worsening of functional abilities. Restrictions on going out and engaging in physical activity – critical for stimulation – negatively influence their cognitive, social and motor functions. Older dementia carers had to cope with a particularly difficult set of issues. In addition to providing the usual level of care, they had to manage a reduction (or no) support from family members or services (curtailed during the pandemic), and also had to factor in their own need to isolate (Cipolletta et al., 2021).

Former carers: carers become 'former carers' (usually) when the cared-for person is permanently admitted to a care home or dies. In the UK, it is estimated that around a third of carers become former carers each year. For many of those whose relative has been admitted to a care home – especially if they are a spouse carer – caring continues post admission albeit in a new form. This role tends to include: visiting their relative regularly; advocating for them; interacting with other residents, relatives and staff; taking part in social events and monitoring the quality of care. They may also continue to offer some of the care they used to provide such as helping their relative with bathing, offering emotional support and managing their money. At a more nuanced level, former carers routinely carry out a range of performative roles such as helping staff to understand the character, life and identity of their relative; this is especially important if the person has dementia (Kirby et al., 2022; Larkin & Milne, 2021).

It is important to recognise that carers tend not to remain static in a single caring role. Many carers move in and out of caring roles over the life course becoming a former carer more than once. For example, a woman may care for her parent and then, some years later, for her husband. This is termed serial caring. Some carers will also care for two or more people simultaneously such as an elderly parent *and* a disabled son or daughter (Larkin, 2009; Larkin et al., 2019).

Family Members Supporting a Relative With a Terminal Illness

Although it is difficult to gauge the exact number of family carers supporting a relative with a 'terminal illness' as the term is variously interpreted, it is currently estimated that between 15% and 20% of carers in the UK are in this situation. The number has grown significantly over the past 20 years. This is as a consequence of three trends: the extension of life amongst those with terminal conditions such as some types of cancer, a growth in the number of older people with life-limiting illnesses such as heart failure, and a preference for community-based care (home or hospice) at the end of life instead of hospital care (Ateş et al., 2018).

Carers of relatives with a terminal illness are mainly female and tend to be spouses/partners or sons or daughters. They are often motivated by a desire to keep caring as long as possible in order to avoid the need for hospital admission or residential care. There is growing recognition of the central role that family carers play in the provision of end-of-life care overall. Studies show that they manage a wide range of responsibilities and fulfil multiple roles (e.g. in addition to personal care they manage symptoms and administer pain relief medication) often without any, or minimal, training. Predictably, caring is very time-consuming and demanding: over half of carers for those with a terminal illness report that they are on duty 24/7. Whilst this may last a few days or months, it can be a role that lasts for years. A carer supporting a relative with a terminal illness is estimated to save the UK economy around £18,000 each year (savings related to not using public services) (Ateş et al., 2018; Morris et al., 2015).

CONCLUDING COMMENTS

Demographic changes means that the number of carers is predicted to increase (Yeandle et al., 2017). For those who are able and willing to offer care it is likely that they will find themselves caring more intensively as a consequence of two factors: the needs of the cared-for population being greater and publicly funded services being in even shorter supply. There are also likely to be more people caring for more than one person; for someone they are not closely related to, e.g. a stepson or stepdaughter; and caring at a distance.

The projected increase in the 'demand' for care is unlikely to match the 'supply' of carers. There are two drivers of reduced supply. One is the trend towards smaller and more dispersed family models: there are simply fewer adult daughters (and sons) to support an elderly parent in any one family. There is also an increase in the number of older people ageing without children (Ray et al., 2015). This is a fundamental challenge for UK society and other developed countries too; a related challenge is protecting those who do provide care from being overburdened.

This chapter has highlighted the extent to which caring can be a source of inequality; both of itself and in terms of being more onerous for some family carers than others. Those groups more profoundly impacted are: women, co-resident carers, dementia carers, older carers and those who are socio-economically disadvantaged. Exploration of the different ways caring can impact on a carer's life, health and well-being is the focus of the next chapter.

3

IMPACT AND CONSEQUENCES OF CARING ON CARERS

INTRODUCTION

It is widely acknowledged that the impact of caring on carers' lives is multi-dimensional, complex and intersectional. Satisfactions and benefits commonly associated with caring include personal growth and enhancing carers' feelings of self-worth, gratification and a sense of 'doing good'. Caring can also deepen the relationship between the carer and the care recipient and help to develop closer relationships with other family members and friends. There may be opportunities for new relationships with paid care staff too (Cheshire-Allen & Calder, 2022; Larkin et al., 2019; Pysklywec et al., 2020). However the positive effects of caring tend to be associated with less intensive levels of care, shorter durations of caring and in contexts where care is offered willingly and without undue pressure (Brimblecombe, et al., 2018a; Whittaker & Gallagher, 2019). Any positive effects also need to be considered alongside the substantive body of evidence about the many adverse consequences in relation to carers' employment, finances, and health and well-being. This chapter explores these consequences on carers in general and for specific groups of carers too (for the sake of consistency, these will be the same groups as in Chapter 2).

As discussed in Chapter 2 becoming a carer is often a gradual process, and caring tends to evolve over time. The impact of caring tends to evolve too over the course of the care trajectory. Care is not a static state; there is also considerable individual variation in experiences of caring. We have attempted to reflect the temporal nature of caring in this chapter as far as we are able. This is a challenge as research tends to capture care at one point in time. We return to the nature of research on caring later in the book.

EMPLOYMENT AND CARING

As explained in Chapter 2, the most recent survey data show that just over half (53%) of family carers are in paid work. Caring responsibilities can intrude into a carer's working life in profound ways: they may be mentally pre-occupied with concerns about care issues and may be regularly interrupted too due to needing to respond to unanticipated events, e.g. an accident, or the failure of a paid carer to arrive as planned. Carers who combine work and caring consistently report 'juggling priorities' (Carers UK, 2019c). Although there is emerging evidence that working carers are less likely to be depressed than non-working carers (O'Neill et al., 2022), there are many studies which identify working carers as experiencing high levels of fatigue and stress and that caring responsibilities have a negative impact upon work roles. For instance, carers may be less able to undertake training or acquire new qualifications, thereby hindering the advancement of their career and compromising promotion opportunities and earning potential (Burr & Colley, 2019; Carers UK, 2019c).

Juggling these challenges can be overwhelming, and without access to support by formal services many carers feel that they have no option other than to reduce their hours or leave employment altogether. Evidence suggests that just over 2.1 million people a year reduce their working hours; carers are more likely to work part time than non-carers. Capacity to remain in work is threatened by care demands. Recent data show that each year 2.6 million people in the UK 'give up work in order to care' with the result that 36% of working-age carers are *not* in work, compared to 23% of non-carers (Carers UK, 2019b; Department for Work and Pensions, 2020; Petrie & Kirkup, 2018). Adults in Wales and Scotland are more likely to have to give up work to care (6% and 7%, respectively) compared with the UK average of 5%. Those in Northern Ireland were less likely to report that 'their work had been negatively affected by caring': 4% compared with 7% overall (Carers UK, 2019b; Centre for Ageing Better, 2021). The longer a carer is out of work, the harder it is to return which has inevitable consequences for carers' future employment prospects and for their current and future earnings.

These patterns were inflated by the pandemic (Carers UK, 2019c); some of those leaving work took retirement earlier than anticipated. It illustrates well the extent to which carers struggle to balance work demands and caring-related demands.

Research also highlights the role played by gender, age and/ or social class. That more women give up work to care has been attributed to the fact that female carers feel a greater sense of obligation to provide care and are more reluctant to ask for support from services than their male counterparts (Burr & Colley, 2019). People aged 45+ are also more likely to both give up work to care and to say that their work had been 'affected negatively' than younger cohorts. This is consistent with the fact that people are most likely to take on caring responsibilities between the ages of 40 and 64 years of age and the fact that those in their 40s and 50s may also be supporting adult sons and daughters.

In relation to social class, there is a greater likelihood that those in lower socio-economic groups have had to give up paid work to provide care than people in higher socio-economic groups. However, the same proportion have been obliged to reduce their working hours to care. In addition to these structural factors disability has been found to play a role; 61% of working-age disabled carers compared to 52% of non-disabled working-age carers gave up work to provide care (Carers, UK, 2019a).

These structural dimensions of caring not only intersect with each other but also with another significant influence on whether carers work full time or only work part time: the number of hours spent caring. As Tables 3.1 and 3.2, respectively, show, family carers who care for 20+ hours a week are 21.9% less likely to be in paid work than non-carers and those who provide 20+ hours of care are 9% more likely to be working part time than non-carers (Petrie & Kirkup, 2018). Contributory factors include: a lack of flexible working arrangements in many workplaces and combining paid work with Carer's Allowance (the main social security benefit for carers: see below). Carers may experience difficulties trying to combine paid work with their caring duties whilst simultaneously satisfying the legal conditions for receipt of this benefit; increases in the National Minimum/Living Wage for example, can push them above the Carer's Allowance earnings limit (Powell et al., 2020).

The negative impact of caring on carers' engagement in employment has implications for the productivity of the economy and for businesses and employers. The resultant increased payment of social security benefits and reduced tax

Table 3.1. Likelihood of Being in Paid Work by Hours of Care.

Hours of Care Per Week	Percentage Difference in Likelihood of Being in Paid Work Compared to Non-Carers
Low hours (fewer than 10 hours)	2.0%
Medium hours (between 10 and 20 hours)	−4.6%
High hours (20 hours or more)	−21.9%

Source: Petrie and Kirkup (2018).

Table 3.2. Likelihood of Working Part-Time by Hours of Care.

Hours of Care	Percentage Difference in Part-Time Work Compared to Non-Carers
Low hours (fewer than 10 hours)	2.9%
Medium hours (between 10 and 20 hours)	3.9%
High hours (20 hours or more)	9.0%

Source: Petrie and Kirkup (2018).

receipts are estimated to constitute a loss to the economy of £2.9 billion per year. The sheer number of employees affected by caring responsibilities means that employers can face unplanned absences and staff recruitment and retention problems. More specifically, the fact that there is a greater likelihood of those aged 45+ giving up work to care means losing employees who are in their prime working years when they are at their most skilled and knowledgeable and in leadership or managerial positions. (Burr & Colley, 2019; Carers UK, 2019c). There is some evidence that these productivity concerns manifest themselves in a risk-averse attitude among employers regarding not recruiting those with caring responsibilities (Powell et al., 2020).

CARERS AND FINANCIAL HARDSHIP

Many carers face very difficult financial situations due to their caring responsibilities; nearly two fifths of carers say that they are struggling to 'make ends meet'. Survey data show the financial hardship results in carers 'cutting back on spending' on essentials, including food and heating (47%) and social activities (64%); drawing down on their savings (44%); and using their bank account overdraft (33%). 21% report being, or having been, in debt as a direct consequence of caring, 15% have fallen into arrears with utility bills and 9% are falling into arrears with their housing costs, i.e. rent or mortgage payments (Carers UK, 2019b; Shooshtari et al., 2017). The pandemic and cost of living crisis have led to a worsening of carers' financial situations generally and have amplified pre-existing debts and money worries (Carers UK, 2021a, 2022b, 2022c).

Some carers are more likely to experience financial hardship and poverty than others. These include carers who have an illness or disability themselves and younger women carers. Overall, 28% of female working-age carers, and 26% of male working-age carers are living in poverty. The gender gap is larger for carers under 35: nearly 40% of young female carers are living in poverty, compared to just over 25% of their male counterparts. Unsurprisingly, length and intensity of caring have been found to be influential too. Those who have been caring for 15 years or more and those who care for more than 35 hours a week are more likely to say that they are struggling (Carers UK, 2019b; Petrie & Kirkup, 2018).

There are significant associations between carers' financial hardship and employment status (Duncan et al., 2020). Loss of earnings, resulting from having to reduce their hours or leave paid work altogether, is a key cause of financial problems. Paradoxically, carers who manage to remain in work earn (on average) £100 pw less than non-carers. The poverty rate for working-age carers is around 25%, compared to around 20% of non-carers. Importantly too, a lower income can adversely impact an individual's pension in terms of reduced accumulation and ineligibility due to earnings below company pension thresholds (Carers UK, 2019c; Centre for Ageing Better, 2021). The employment-related consequences of caring are therefore strongly linked to financial hardship in the present and in the future.

Carers also need to contend with care-related expenditures; direct costs related to caring that would not have been incurred otherwise. These include: purchasing specialised aids and devices; additional laundry demands (linked to incontinence); extra heating due to being at home for more hours and/or to support a health condition; higher telephone bills because of issues such as arranging support, sorting out health appointments and travel costs; and paying for care services.

All of these costs may compromise carers' ability to meet their own expenses and reduce their opportunities to save and invest; balancing the books may simply be impossible for some low-income families, made worse by COVID and the 2022 cost of living crisis (Carers UK, 2022b, 2022c; Duncan et al., 2020; Powell et al., 2020).

Carer's Allowance can be a vital source of support in terms of paying bills, meeting the extra costs of caring and providing a credit towards state pensions and other contributory benefits. However, although it is not means tested many carers – even when they care full time – are not eligible because of entitlement conditions (namely an earnings limit and exclusion because of being in full-time education and being in receipt of certain other benefits, including a State Pension). Furthermore, it is the lowest non-means tested income replacement of all benefits in the UK – currently £69.70 a week (2022–2023) and those who *do* qualify find that it is inadequate. Over half of carers who are receiving Carer's Allowance (53%) 'struggle to cope financially' (Carers UK, 2019b, 2021a). The eligibility criteria used, and the low level of the payment, means that the benefit does *not* prevent financial hardship amongst carers, one of its purported aims.

HEALTH AND WELL-BEING

Over half (52%) of carers feel 'stressed' about their financial situation. That being a carer is also physically and psychologically demanding means that caring, particularly intensive caring, can be very stressful (Carers UK, 2021a; Xu et al., 2021). The pandemic elevated carers' anxiety levels. Whilst this has been mainly attributed to increased caring burden and financial costs (Abbasi-Shavazi et al., 2022; Carers UK,

2020a), carers also faced the additional challenge of protecting the person they care for from COVID. Issues included conflict between carers and their relative over the interpretation of the guidance issued, adapting and transitioning to different ways of working (i.e. online and homeworking) and caring with depleted resources (Cipolletta et al., 2021; Lafferty et al., 2022).

Whether they work or not, many carers, especially those caring for more than 20 hours per week, often have very limited free time; a situation also exacerbated by the pandemic. For instance, they do not have time for 'healthy living', such as exercising, maintaining a balanced diet and getting sufficient sleep. Pressures on their time can also lead to carers being unable to attend their own medical appointments or having to delay or even cancel an operation or treatment because of caring responsibilities (Powell et al., 2020). In addition, they have to sacrifice their personal and social life. There is little time, energy and money to take breaks, pursue an interest, invest in friendships or engage in leisure and social activities. Recent research shows that 80% of carers report 'feeling lonely or isolated' as a result of a diminution of their relationships with others; this rate is seven times higher than that of the general population (Larkin et al., 2019). It is a particularly pronounced issue for female and LGBTQ+ carers. For example, in 2020, 93% of female carers reported feeling lonely and isolated compared to 87% of male carers; 63% of LGBTQ+ carers reported feeling lonely and isolated compared to 52% of heterosexual carers (Carers UK, 2021b).

There are a number of other under-researched and more hidden experiences which can deepen carers' sense of isolation and loneliness. One of the most widely reported is lack of 'positive social recognition': recognising and valuing what carers do (Moore & Gillespie, 2014). A second is limited acknowledgement of the physical, emotional, verbal or sexual coercion and/or aggression from the person they care for. Whether this behaviour is intentional or unintentional or incidental or systematic, it is physically and/or psychologically harmful; carers often feel frightened and vulnerable (Isham et al., 2020). Studies show that carers are disinclined to disclose what is happening to them because they fear their relative being 'removed' to a care home or that they would be condemned for 'not coping'. This fear can lead to carers adopting defensive coping strategies, e.g. emotional containment and minimisation of contact with family, friends and services. This deepens carers' level of social isolation. There is also a reluctance to believe the carer and/or a resistance to hearing what they are reporting. Many sons or daughters, for example, cannot accept that their much-loved dad is behaving aggressively. Rather than accepting this, they will 'deny' it or construct it as 'much less usual' than their mother is reporting. Most of us have difficulty understanding, let alone accepting, the profoundly negative impacts of caring especially when it contradicts our own perceptions of what care 'should be like'. It also contradicts the public and policy narrative about family care being wholly positive and virtuous and all carers being competent at providing care (Isham et al., 2020; Spencer et al., 2019).

All of the above factors – stress, anxiety, loneliness, social isolation, reduced opportunities for healthy living and to have a 'life outside of caring' – inevitably compromise carers' quality of life and health and well-being. This is further amplified when they feel they have little, or no, choice about undertaking the role (Al-Janabi et al., 2018; Moore & Gillespie, 2014). On average carers rate their 'general happiness' as 15% lower than the general population (NHS Digital, 2019). Carers are also 50% more likely to report poor 'physical and psychological well-being' than people without caring responsibilities (Carers UK, 2019a; Powell et al., 2020).

Furthermore, recent research shows that caring can nega-tively, and permanently, alter immunity and stress hormones. This not only leaves carers more vulnerable to becoming ill (such as developing chronic illness, getting COVID) but also means carers face an increased risk of future illness or disability – by up to 33% – irrespective of whether, or when, they stop caring (Gallagher & Bennett, 2021).

Let's take a closer look at the available data. In 2019, 63% of carers had at least one long-term health condition, disability or illness compared to 50% of non-carers (Ipsos Mori, 2021) and over a quarter (27%) were in receipt of Disability Living Allowance[1] (Carers UK, 2019b). Physical health issues include musculoskeletal and back problems (often linked to the physical tasks of caring such as moving and handling, bathing and dressing), heart disease, exhaus-tion, skin disorders and infections, arthritis, sciatica, high blood pressure, asthma, hernias and dental issues. Some carers report multiple health problems (Larkin & Milne, 2014; NHS Digital, 2019). In terms of psychological morbidity carers are nearly twice as likely to suffer from depression and anxiety than non-carers (Carers UK, 2019a). There is also an emerging body of international evidence which suggests that

---

1 This is now being replaced by Personal Independence Payment (PIP) but the criteria were:

- Having had specific care and/or mobility needs for at least three months before claiming Allowance and expecting to have them for at least six months after.
- Care needs were defined as needing help with/being supervised when, getting dressed, going to the toilet or cooking a main meal
- A person was deemed to have mobility needs if they have a physical or mental disability which means that they walk with difficulty, cannot walk, cannot walk outdoors or on an unfamiliar route without help from someone else most of the time.

carers may be a high-risk group for suicide (O'Dwyer et al., 2021).

It is important to recognise that a number of these issues may precede caring, or not be linked to it at all. For example, some of those who become carers may have pre-existing disabilities or long-term health conditions. In 2019, 23% of carers considered themselves to have a disability *before* they started caring (Carers UK, 2019b; Milne, 2020). As noted in Chapter 2, this is likely to be a particular issue for the third of carers who are aged 65+. However useful data on the impact of caring on carers' health and well-being are, they do not capture any multiplier effect on carers with pre-existing health problems. This is an important deficit to address.

A number of groups of carers are at particular risk of poor health outcomes. These include female carers, co-resident carers, carers looking after disabled children under the age of 18 years, those who provide more than 50 hours of care per week, older carers and those who have been caring for over 15 years (Carers UK, 2019a; Powell et al., 2020). There is also some evidence that the proportion of carers reporting negative effects of caring on their health is increasing year on year (NHS Digital, 2019). The pandemic had a further detrimental impact; 69% of carers reported that their mental health had worsened and 64% that their physical health has deteriorated (Carers UK, 2021b; Whitley et al., 2021). Despite a great deal of evidence about carers' health and well-being being profoundly negatively affected by caring, carers consistently report that they feel their health care needs are *not* being met (Public Health England, 2021). This is an issue which we return to later in the book.

IMPACT OF CARING ON SPECIFIC
CARER POPULATIONS

In this section we are going to take a closer look at the impacts of caring on a number of the carer populations explored in Chapter 2. Differences and variations are highlighted.

BAME Carers

Although there is relatively little research in this area, there is evidence that BAME carers are likely to suffer greater ill-health than their white counterparts. Whilst this has been attributed to the fact that they provide disproportionately more care and are more likely to be obliged to give up paid employment, structural issues also play a role. There are additional barriers relating to discrimination, culture, language and socio-economic disadvantage. A number of BAME communities are at higher risk of: unemployment (e.g. Black African Caribbean and South Asian communities); financial issues because of low incomes or poverty (particularly Pakistani and Bangladeshi communities); social exclusion and ill-health (Carers UK, 2011; Nair et al., 2022).

Sandwich Carers

Evidence suggests that sandwich carers are more likely to struggle financially, feel less satisfied with life and report symptoms of mental ill-health compared with the general population. Indeed almost 27% of sandwich carers show symptoms of common mental health problems, including depression and anxiety (Carers UK, 2019a; Embracing Carers, 2021). This is a gender issue as more women than men are sandwich carers. That the peak age for sandwich caring for women also coincides with when many women are at the peak of their careers underscores a number of the issues discussed earlier in relationship to compromised career progression and financial disadvantage (Oldridge & Larkin, 2020).

Young Carers

As noted in Chapter 2, young carers often experience a number of disadvantages. Closer examination of the evidence shows that whilst individual young carers are affected in different ways, there are a number of commonalities (Carers UK, 2019b). On the positive side, caring can be rewarding for young carers; it is routinely associated with a range of positive emotional and psychological benefits including happiness, increased self-esteem, self-worth, satisfaction, capacity to deal with challenges, a sense of maturity and a strong 'moral consciousness' in that they see moral value in the caring role (Boyle, 2020; Larkin et al., 2019). Nonetheless care responsibilities can have significant and adverse long-term effects on young carers' lives, a number of which are illustrated in Sam's story below.

Case Study: Sam's Story

Sam's brother, Max, was born with a condition known as foetal valproate syndrome, that includes hypermobility, visual impairment and autism. When Sam's father left the family home Sam was only six years old but immediately started helping his mother care for Max. As the brothers had to share a bedroom, Sam was often disturbed at night and his constant tiredness meant his schoolwork suffered. At secondary school he was often

(Continued)

bullied and became withdrawn, spending most of the time out of class on his own. He found it difficult to develop friendships and was unable to socialise or even spend time on his own at home because of Max's behaviour. His mother's reliance on his support meant he had to miss days at school and did not join in with after-school activities as he had to get home to help with Max. However, his relationship with his mother was becoming increasingly strained because they were both under enormous stress and were prone to uncontrolled aggressive outbursts.

When it came to GCSEs he was finding it really hard to keep up with coursework because of his inability to concentrate and repeated absences from school. As a result, he was put back by a year and became even more isolated from his peer group. There were several gangs on his estate. When approached by a member of one of these gangs on the way home from school he decided to meet with them for an hour every so often in the evenings when he could get away from home without too many questions being asked. He was soon drawn into the gang's petty criminal activities because he wanted to be accepted by his peers and was lonely. It was not long before he was caught with some of the other members shoplifting at the local 24-hour supermarket....

Caring tends to have a more profound impact on a young carer's life when care responsibilities are very demanding, of two years or more duration, and access to formal support is limited or non-existent. Unsurprisingly, the health and well-being of young carers is poorer than their peers. Recent studies have found that 40% of young carers report mental health problems as a direct result of caring (James, 2019; Lewis et al., 2023); these include anxiety, distress, depression, fatigue and 'feelings of anger'. Young carers also tend to be more socially isolated (especially during the pandemic when 80% of young carers reported this), stigmatised and unsupported by services; they feel they are missing out on enjoying their childhood and on developing friendships with their peers (Cheesbrough et al., 2017; Gallagher et al., 2022; Powell et al., 2020). Young carers who are lonely and isolated are particularly vulnerable to hidden harm, and developing unhealthy or actively dangerous coping mechanisms such as self-harm, substance misuse and offending behaviour (Jacklin, 2021; Lewis et al., 2023).

As Sam's story shows, caring responsibilities have implications for young carers' education too. Compared to their peers, there is a greater probability that they will regularly be absent from, or late for, school (see Fig. 3.1), be unable to complete their homework, and struggle to concentrate due to tiredness, even falling asleep whilst at school (see Fig. 3.2). For these reasons, young carers have significantly lower educational attainment at GCSE level and gain fewer qualifications than their peers. This all has consequences for their post-compulsory education, training and employment opportunities, reflected in the fact that young carers aged 16–19 are more likely than their peers to not be in education, training or employment (NEET). Inevitably such consequences jeopardise their career opportunities, earning potential and future prospects in adult life (Hounsell, 2013; Powell et al., 2020).

The extent to which young carers are disadvantaged by their social and cultural backgrounds was discussed in Chapter 2. Arguably such disadvantages would exist whether they were caring or not, but it seems fair to assume that caring magnifies the impact of pre-existing adversities. Another

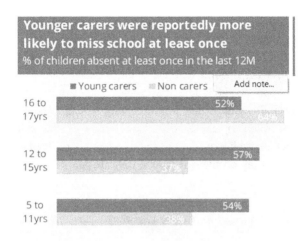

Source: Powell et al. (2020).

Fig. 3.1. Young Carers' School Absences.

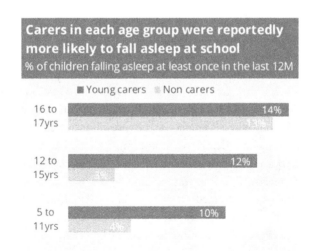

Source: Powell et al. (2020).

Fig. 3.2. Young Carers and Falling Asleep at School.

factor that merits consideration when interpreting the evidence is how it has been gathered. Collecting information from *both* the cared-for person (usually a parent) and young carer has been found to build a much fuller picture of the caring context including the range and nature of care responsibilities and their impact on the young person's life (Cheesbrough et al., 2017). This reinforces the call for research that takes account of the wider family or dyad rather than focussing on the carer alone (see Chapter 5).

Older Carers

In contrast to the relatively large volume of research on young carers, there are few studies which focus exclusively on older carers (Greenwood et al., 2019). The small body of work that does exist identifies that older carers are at a higher risk of experiencing a range of health problems than other groups of adult carers. Overall, 65% have long-term health problems. Although age-related health conditions are inevitably contributory factors, older carers' health problems are known to be caused, and/or exacerbated by, caring responsibilities especially if they are intensive and/or long term. These include: cardiac problems, back issues/pain, hypertension, sleep problems, strain, fatigue, anxiety and depression. Indeed 40% of older carers have depressive symptoms, attributable, in part at least, to a number of care-related risks. These include: isolation, loneliness, feeling trapped and being both emotionally and physically drained (Larkin et al., 2019; Maun et al., 2020). That they support relatives with more complex needs and are expected to do more in terms of care tasks with no or very limited input from services means that their health problems are likely to worsen over time. Many older carers also worry about the future when they may no longer be able to provide care due to their own ill-health or death (Greenwood et al., 2019). This has been found to be a major concern for older parents of middle-aged sons or daughters with learning disabilities (Mahon et al., 2019).

Older carers are typically living on a reduced or fixed income as most are retired. Care-related expenditure (referred to above) tends to be higher for older carers because of the needs of the cared-for person. In addition, they may have to pay for care services or aids to help them cope, e.g. incontinence equipment, a cleaner or home carer. This means they are also at risk of falling into poverty.

Dementia Carers

That older carers are increasingly supporting people living with dementia was discussed in Chapter 2. The fact that the many challenges faced by dementia carers were heightened during the pandemic was also addressed. As caring for someone with dementia is one of the most difficult and demanding caring roles, it is linked to some of the worst health outcomes for carers (Greenwood & Smith, 2019).

In addition to the health and financial problems experienced by older carers generally, dementia carers have a greater likelihood of: feeling restricted and trapped because they are unable to leave their relative; decreased social connectedness as friends may be reluctant to visit; being exposed to stigma; strained relationships in the wider family; daily conflicts with the person arising from dementia-related symptoms; and aggression or abuse by the person living with dementia. Spousal carers, in particular, also struggle to cope with the loss of a shared life course, memories and experiences, and the reduced companionship and emotional connectedness with their partner (Milne, 2020).

An increasing number of studies have explored carers' positive experiences in supporting a relative with dementia. These have been identified as: role satisfaction, reciprocity, emotional rewards, personal growth, competence and feeling 'they were making a difference' and 'doing their duty'. Work adopting a dyadic lens has been particularly useful in this area of carer research (Lloyd et al., 2016; Pysklywec et al., 2020; Quinn et al., 2022).

Former Carers

Research that has been done on former carers consistently shows that they are exposed to a range of disadvantages arising from their caring experiences. These have been referred to as the 'legacies of caring' and are particularly profound for those who have cared over the long term and intensively (Larkin, 2009; Larkin & Milne, 2017).

Depleted savings, debt, being in arrears, lack of income due to working reduced hours/giving up work to care and reduced retirement income all mean that many carers are left with a negative financial legacy. That carers lose their carer-related benefits once 'active' caring ends compounds the situation. Opportunities to address financial losses post-caring can be very limited even for those of working age; work-related skills and social networks lost during caring can damage prospects of returning to a pre-caring job or embarking on a new career post-caring (Cavaye & Watts, 2018; Cronin et al., 2015).

Contraction of social networks and lower levels of social activity during caring is linked to another legacy of caring, social isolation. The well-documented physical and psychological health problems linked with caring often persist into, and may worsen, post-caring. For example, back pain, exhaustion, skin disorders, infections, arthritis, high blood pressure, cardiac problems and social isolation. New health issues that develop after caring ends include sleep and eating problems and increased alcohol consumption (Cronin et al., 2015; Larkin & Milne, 2017).

The degree to which these legacies are experienced depends on a number of variables. For example, more problematic caring experiences, such as those which involved a strained relationship with the cared-for person, are linked to lower levels of well-being amongst former carers. A further influence on the legacies of caring is bereavement. This can be more challenging for carers than non-carers and have longer-term emotional consequences. One explanation is that carers – unlike those whose relatives die without needing family care – often experience many years of 'anticipatory loss' (i.e. loss of freedom and hopes for the future) linked to a deterioration in the care recipient's health. This process can give rise to a multitude of complex emotions, both during caring and after death (Larkin & Milne, 2021).

Family Members Supporting a Relative With a Terminal Illness

A number of studies highlight the rewards of caring for a relative who is terminally ill. These include the positive impact on self-esteem and the facilitation of a close bond with the dying person. For example, an adult son or daughter may be able to spend more time with a parent than they may have done for many years. Being able to remain at home is emphasised in research; it allows carers to maintain a normal routine with their relative for as long as possible. It also offers a greater chance of being able to provide a sense of peace and dignity at the actual point of death (Ateş et al., 2018).

However, carers of people who are terminally ill often experience high levels of burden, particularly as the illness worsens. Whilst the general unpreparedness of family carers to cope with the overwhelming demands they have to face is a contributory factor, so too are the physical and mental strains involved in this type of caring. These strains are, partly, a product of sleep deprivation, isolation, anxiety, stress and distress. Being the sole carer and feeling that their efforts are not acknowledged by paid carers have been identified as exacerbating these impacts, as has carers' suspension of control over their own health, needs and diet in order to provide the best possible quality of care to their relative. Although it has been suggested that the ability to maintain a normal life and engagement with activities may decrease the family carer's vulnerability and protect against fatigue and burnout, further research on this issue is required (Ateş et al., 2018; Morris et al., 2015).

CONCLUDING COMMENTS

This chapter has demonstrated that the links between caring and carer outcomes vary significantly in both depth and nature. Negative outcomes can be mediated, or amplified, by a wide range of factors, e.g. number of hours spent caring, the care relationship, the type of care required, age, family support and level of income. However, unravelling the interaction between positive and negative aspects of caring and the direction and strength of effect(s) is inherently problematic. The fact that caring is a journey that shifts over time is a challenge to capture. Knowledge about the impact and consequences of caring is very dependent on the nature and extent of available research. The fact that research tends to adopt a particular paradigmatic lens on care and caring is an issue we reflect on later in the book.

Chapter 3 also underscores a key theme explored in Chapter 2: namely that caring *of itself* can be a source of inequality. Caring tends to exacerbate existing inequalities relating to age, gender and socio-economic status (and others); it also creates new ones such as additional financial demands and physical and mental health challenges. The fact that inequalities are life course issues and caring is embedded in a life course raises questions about how we understand and explore caring. The outbreak of COVID served to increase public awareness of carers' lives and roles, and growing evidence about the extent of the inequalities they face has led to calls for family care to be considered a social determinant of health (Public Health England, 2021).

The impact of caring intersects strongly with one of the key sources of inequality and unevenness for carers – access to formal care and support. It is to policy, services and support for carers that we now turn in Chapter 4.

4

SUPPORTING CARERS

INTRODUCTION

As a consequence of changing family models, geographical mobility and more people ageing without children, many carers find themselves with no one nearby who can help them manage the demands of caring. Local support networks, made up of extended family members, are increasingly rare. Even when such networks do exist, carers report not being able to rely on relatives and friends as they have their own families, jobs and caring responsibilities. Despite prominent policy claims about the importance of 'recognising and supporting carers', promoting their rights to 'live a life outside caring' and to 'have their needs met' by services, evidence suggests that many carers simply do not receive the support from services they need (Larkin & Milne, 2014).

The many impacts of caring, their persistence and recent amplification due to austerity and COVID, combine with limited access to support to compromise the capacity of many carers to provide the quality of care they would wish. Manthorpe and Illiffe (2016) argue that cutbacks in services have become unjustly framed as a 'moral failure on the part of family carers' who may be accused of being 'abusive or neglectful' when they slip up or make a mistake due to 'exhaustion or despair' (p. 22). Insufficient support can also lead to carer breakdown. Six in ten British carers report that they 'have been pushed to breaking point'; the number of cases of carer breakdown is also rising (Association of Directors of Adult Social Services (ADASS), 2022; Butt, 2020). An increasing number of carers need to be admitted to hospital; sometimes they may be admitted alongside their relative. Unless plans have been put in place (which is rare), family members, social care services and the NHS are routinely left scrambling to put in place emergency care arrangements. Not only does this cause disruption and distress for the person needing care, but it is extremely costly for public services, including the NHS. Crises can also lead to older or disabled relatives being admitted to a care home despite neither they, nor their carer, wanting this outcome (Carers UK, 2014, 2021b). The number of people being admitted to a care home directly from hospital has increased in the last decade; one of the key reasons is carer breakdown.

Not only is effectively supporting carers a matter of social justice (see Chapter 6), but as each family carer is thought to save the UK economy around £20,000+ per year (ADASS, 2022) there are economic incentives to ensuring that family carers are appropriately supported. This chapter will outline carer-related policy and support in the UK and provide an analysis of the outcomes for carers generally and also for a number of the carer populations we have been focussing on in Chapters 2 and 3.

CARER-RELATED POLICES OVER THE LAST TWENTY YEARS

Since the 1980s national carers organisations, such as Carers UK[1] and Carers Trust,[2] have worked tirelessly to raise awareness of the central importance of unpaid care to the fabric of social, family and economic life in the UK. In the context of ever-growing public support for carers, they have also expanded the reach of their campaigning activities to address a range of issues relevant to carers' lives such as poverty and employment rights (Teahan et al., 2021). Their efforts, and those of policy makers, are reflected in the development of a number of key policies and strategies to support carers across the four nations of the UK.

Table 4.1 provides an overview of these policies and strategies, starting with the 1995 Carers (Recognition and Services) Act. Whilst not intended to be fully comprehensive, it does convey the sheer number and range of carer-related policies. The Table also includes a number of cross-cutting laws and policies that affect carers.

Analysis of the policy framework(s) highlights developments in six broad areas. These are discussed below. Reference will made to policies and strategies in Table 4.1 in this section and throughout the rest of the chapter.

---

1 Carers UK is the national membership charity for unpaid carers. Together with their members they campaign to make life better for carers and strive to realise their vision of a society that recognises, values and supports carers for the huge contribution they make to families and communities, https://www.carersuk.org/.

2 The Carers Trust is a charity which works with a unique network of partner organisations, independently managed Carers' Centres and young carers services to help carers with the challenges of their caring roles. The Trust is the largest provider of comprehensive carers support services in the UK, https://carers.org/.

Table 4.1. Policies and Strategies to Support Unpaid Carers in the UK.

	England	Scotland	Wales	Northern Ireland
1995	Carers (Recognition and Services) Act	Carers (Recognition and Services) Act	Carers (Recognition and Services) Act	
1999	'Caring for Carers' Strategy	Scottish Strategy for Carers		
2000	Carers and Disabled Children Act		Caring about Carers: Carers Strategy in Wales Implementation Plan Carers and Disabled Children Act	
2002		Community Care and Health (Scotland) Act		Carers Strategy Carers and Direct Payments (Northern Ireland) Act Valuing Carers: A strategy for Carers in Northern Ireland
2004	Carers (Equal Opportunities) Act		Carers (Equal Opportunities) Act	
2006	Children and Families Act			Caring for Carers
2006		Work and Families Act*		
2007		Pensions Act*		
2008	Strategy: Carers at the heart of twenty-first century families and communities.			
2009				Review of the support provision for carers

	Recognised Valued and Supported: next steps for the carers strategy	Caring Together: the carers strategy for Scotland 2010–2015	Carers Strategies (Wales) Measure	
2010	Recognised Valued and Supported: next steps for the carers strategy	Caring Together: the carers strategy for Scotland 2010–2015	Carers Strategies (Wales) Measure	
2010		Equality Act**		
2013		Social Care (Self-Directed Support) Act		
2014	Care Act Children and Families Act		Social Services and Well-being (Wales) Act	Transforming Your Palliative and End of Life Care Update
2015		Palliative and end-of-life care: strategic framework for action		
2016		Carers (Scotland) Act		Expert Advisory Panel on Adult Care and Support
2017			Palliative and end-of-life care delivery plan	
2018	Carers Action Plan 2018–2020: Support carers today			
2020	National Institute for Health and Care Excellence (NICE) 'Guidelines for supporting unpaid adult carers'**			
2021	Ambitions for Palliative and End of Life Care: a national framework for local action 2021–2026		Strategy for unpaid carers Wales	
2022	Health and Care Act			Reform of Adult Social Care consultation paper

*These apply across the whole of the UK.

**Act applies to Great Britain.

Source: Adapted from Lloyd's book (with authors' permission) (2023).

BENEFITS FOR CARERS

Carers are entitled to a range of benefits. The main cash benefits are the Carer's Allowance (non-means tested and non-contributory) and the Carer Premium (payable with means-tested benefits). Universal Credit also includes a carer element which mirrors the carer premium (worth £168.81 a month in 2022/2023). Box 4.1 provides a comprehensive summary of Carer's Allowance and its entitlement conditions (noted in Chapter 3). Details of the Carer Premium are set out in Box 4.2.

Box 4.1

Carer's Allowance

Carer's Allowance is a benefit for people who are giving regular and substantial care to disabled people. It is a taxable benefit and forms part of claimant's taxable income.

It is payable if a carer:

- is aged 16 or over

- is not in full time education

- is not studying for 21 hours a week or more

- spends at least 35 hours a week caring for a disabled person

- does not earn more than £132 a week (the earnings threshold for Carer's Allowance in 2022) from employment or self-employment after deductions such as income tax, National Insurance and half of your pension contributions

(Continued)

- is not subject to immigration control (that would stop you getting benefits)

- has been in England, Scotland or Wales for at least 2 of the last 3 years (this does not apply if you're a refugee or have humanitarian protection status)

- normally lives in England, Scotland or Wales, or you live abroad as a member of the armed forces (you might still be eligible if you're moving to or already living in an EEA country or Switzerland)

The person being cared for must already be in receipt of one or more of these benefits:

- Personal Independence Payment – daily living component

- Disability Living Allowance – the middle or highest care rate

- Attendance Allowance

- Constant Attendance Allowance at or above the normal maximum rate with an Industrial Injuries Disablement Benefit

- Constant Attendance Allowance at the basic (full day) rate with a War Disablement Pension

- Armed Forces Independence Payment

- Child Disability Payment – the middle or highest care rate

(Continued)

(*Continued*)

- Adult Disability Payment – daily living component

Carer's Allowance is not paid during breaks in care and is either not paid or reduced if a claimant is in receipt of a number of other benefits including:

- state retirement pension

- contributory Employment Support Allowance (ESA)

- contribution-based Job Seekers Allowance (JSA)

- Maternity Allowance

If a carer's Carer's Allowance is either the same as, or less than, the other benefit, he/she will get the other benefit rather than Carer's Allowance. Should the other benefit be less than his/her Carer's Allowance, the carer will receive the other benefit and the balance of the Carer's Allowance on top.

Source: *Adapted from Carer's Allowance - Citizens Advice* and *Carer's Allowance: How it works - GOV.UK (www.gov.uk).*

There are variations in the payment of Carer's Allowance across the devolved nations. For example, in 2020 the Scottish Government introduced an additional Carer's Allowance Supplement beyond the base level of Carer's Allowance backdated to April 2018, paid twice yearly (in June and December). In 2022 this supplement was £245.70. The increase does not affect other benefits, including Income Support, tax credits and Universal Credit.

Box 4.2

Carer Premium

The Carer Premium (also known as the Carer Addition and the Carer Element, depending on which benefit is being claimed) is an additional amount of money paid on top of other means-tested benefits a carer might already be claiming. These are:

- Universal Credit (UC)

- Income Support

- Jobseeker's Allowance (JSA) – income-related

- Employment Support Allowance (ESA) – income-related

- Housing Benefit

- Pension Credit

- Tax Credits (Child and Working)

- Council Tax Support

When a carer does not claim Carer's Allowance but is in receipt of Carer Premium, the person they are caring for cannot get the following added to their qualifying benefit:

- Severe Disability Premium or

- Severe Disability Addition

Source: *Adapted from Carer's Allowance: How it works - GOV.UK (www.gov.uk) and Carers UK (2021b).*

SERVICES AND SUPPORT

Local authorities provide access to publicly funded social care to people with care and support needs and their family carers. They employ eligibility criteria to ensure services are targeted on those 'in greatest need'. These criteria have been raised in response to a rolling back of the welfare state, and more recently, austerity.

'Carer needs assessments' were introduced by the Carers (Recognition and Services) Act, 1995. At this time, carers were only eligible for an assessment if they were 'providing a substantial amount of care on a regular basis'. The 2014 Care Act changed this; all carers are now entitled to a 'statutory assessment of need' from their local authority regardless of the quantity of care they provide. Some local authorities do their own carers assessments in-house whilst others have commissioned assessments from third-sector carers organisations. The needs assessment is expected to consider factors such as: the carer's willingness to provide care, the impact of their own health and support needs on their ability to provide care, and the extent to which the provision of support could contribute to carer well-being and employment, educational and/or health related outcomes.

Section 20 of the Care Act, 2014, places a duty on local authorities to provide services to all (adult) carers in their area who meet national eligibility criteria.[3] Even when the criteria are

---

3 A carer is deemed to have eligible needs if they meet all the following criteria:

- Do your needs arise because you are providing necessary care for an adult?
- Do these needs mean you are unable to achieve a range of tasks or 'outcomes' such as managing your own nutrition, taking part in work, training or education, maintaining a habitable and safe home?
- As a result of this, is there likely to be a significant impact on your well-being?

not met, local authorities have discretionary powers – but not a duty – to provide support. Where support is provided, a local authority must prepare a 'care and support plan' for each carer outlining how their needs are going to be met. If the local authority wishes to charge a carer for the provision of support (whether eligible or not), it must carry out a financial assessment of what they can afford to pay (i.e. a means test). The person they care for may also be eligible to receive care and support services in their own right. They (usually) receive a separate assessment of need and care and support plan, although there is a move towards assessing the needs of the carer *and* cared-for person jointly as a unit or dyad (Rand et al., 2022).

Carer Health and Well-Being

The Government has emphasised the importance of (1) the routine identification of carers and (2) integrated care in meeting carers' health and well-being needs. This is reflected in NHS England's Commitment to Carers programme (launched in 2014) and the publication of an 'integrated approach to identifying and assessing carer health and well-being' in 2016 (NHS England, 2014). The latter set out principles for joint working between organisations in order to improve the identification and assessment of carers in primary care; provide integrated packages of care to support carers' physical and mental health needs; and give carers choices about how support is delivered. The ongoing commitment to improve how the NHS identifies carers, and to better address their health needs, is also a key feature of the Carers Action Plan 2018–2020.

The *National Institute for Health and Care Excellence* (NICE) guidelines for 'Supporting adult carers' (2020) extends this commitment. It sets out the responsibilities of NHS organisations (such as GPs, pharmacists and hospitals) and local authorities to identify, support and involve adult carers when assessing and planning services for adults with care and support needs. Other initiatives have focussed on interventions to improve carer health and well-being such as social prescribing (for example, to connect people to community groups and agencies for practical and emotional support) and the provision of carers' breaks.

Young Carers

The Children and Families Act, 2014, gave carers under the age of 18 (in England) the same right to a needs assessment as adult carers, including an assessment of the 'appropriateness' of the caring responsibilities the child is undertaking. Unlike assessments provided for adult carers, there are no national eligibility criteria for provision of services; following a young carer's assessment, local authorities have discretion about whether to provide support for the young person or not.

In terms of available support, level and types of service(s) vary by area. Some schools offer a counselling service for young carers. In England, if a young carer is entitled to free school meals, s/he may also be eligible for Pupil Premium funding; this is extra funding for schools to support the education of 'disadvantaged children'. This funding goes directly to a young carer's school. In 2019 it was estimated that 60% of carers aged 14–16 years were eligible for free school meals. This suggests that many young carers are eligible for Pupil Premium funding.

There are also a number of support programmes, resources and services targeted at young carers. An example is the 'Young carers in schools' programme, run jointly by Carers Trust and The Children's Society.[4] This initiative works with schools

4 https://www.childrenssociety.org.uk/

across England and Wales to share good practice, provide training and support, increase identification of young carers and improve engagement. In Scotland, carers aged 11–18 years are provided with a 'Young carers package' in recognition of their role. This includes digital vouchers, access to subscriptions and exclusive discount opportunities at selected shops. Some local authorities commission specific services. For example, one County Council commissioned a young carers service to provide assessments, signposting, one to one support, monthly youth clubs and summer holiday activities. It also delivered a Young Carer Ambassador Programme, details of which are set out in Box 4.3.

Box 4.3

Young Carer Ambassador Programme

Wovenshire Council's 'Young Carer Ambassador Programme' offers up to sixty 10- to 18-year old carers a place on one of four performing arts workshops held throughout the year, focussing on improving communication, public speaking and presentation skills, and ultimately supporting young people to develop the skills that employers look for. The project also aims to encourage a number of young people to become Young Carer Ambassadors following involvement in one of the workshops. This role will see them co-deliver assemblies at their schools – alongside the Wovenshire Young Carers Education Link Worker – where they share their story of being a carer. They are also practicing skills in public speaking, presentation and communication.

The health and well-being of young carers has been the subject of a number of initiatives introduced by NHS England. One such initiative is the establishment of the Young Carers Health Champion Programme. This involves young carers in devising ways of supporting health literacy and promoting the health and well-being of young carers. Another is a voluntary scheme to encourage GP practices to identify and support children and young people providing care for family members.

Young carers (aged 16–19) in further education may be entitled to a discretionary bursary which is intended to remove barriers to learning. However, young people with caring responsibilities are reluctant to self-identify because of fear of being stigmatised (See Chapter 3). Although Carer's Allowance can be claimed from the age of 16, those in full-time education are excluded from claiming (see Box 4.1). In 2019, as part of their broader package of support for young carers, the Scottish Government introduced an annual Young Carer Grant – £326.65 in 2022 – payable to people aged 16–18 who 'provide at least 16 hours of care a week to a person receiving a qualifying disability benefit, but who do not qualify for Carer's Allowance'.

Carers and Higher Education

Carers are now one of the priority groups for widening participation[5] within Higher Education. Many universities

---

5 Widening participation refers to the work done in education to increase the number of young people entering higher education, and more specifically increasing the proportion of these students who are from under-represented groups.

and colleges have adopted carers policies to support students who are carers as part of their equality agenda. These policies aim to accommodate the additional challenges a student with caring responsibilities has whilst simultaneously ensuring these do not compromise academic standards. They typically include:

- *academic help*: for example – flexible deadlines, help with workload management, or priority access to academic or career opportunities (e.g. internships)

- *financial support* in the form of a scholarship, grant or bursary

- *health and well-being support*: as well as support services on campus, some universities and colleges offer induction days over the summer to help student carers settle in and give them the chance to discuss their support needs ahead of the start of term

- *carer passports*: these are a form of 'carer ID' and mean that student carers can access help and support without having to share their story multiple times with different staff across the university

One of the largest carers organisations – *Carers Trust* – have been very active in promoting support for young carers and young adult carers and have published a guidance document to help universities formulate carer policies that will help student carers access, and succeed in, Higher Education. Fig. 4.1 is a model for working with student carers that *Carers Trust* has developed; it usefully illustrates the way support for student carers can be delivered.

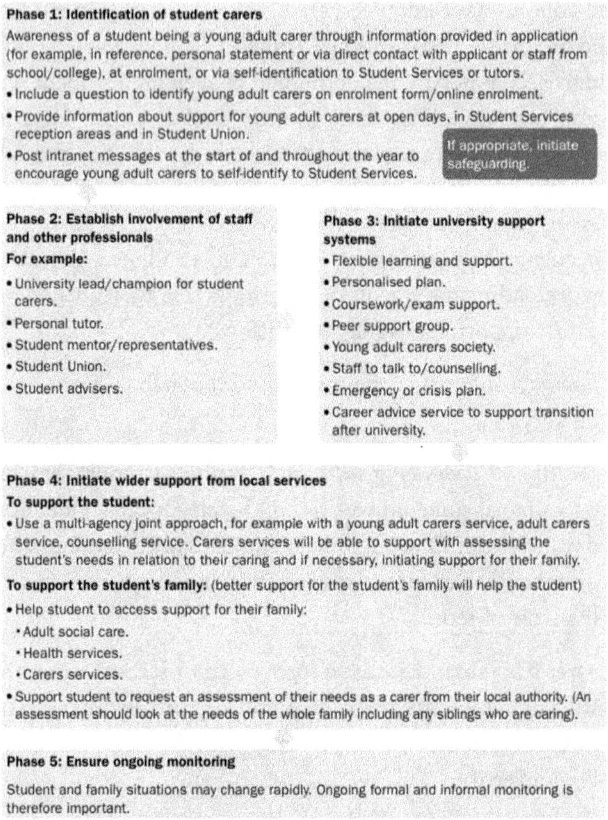

Phase 1: Identification of student carers

Awareness of a student being a young adult carer through information provided in application (for example, in reference, personal statement or via direct contact with applicant or staff from school/college), at enrolment, or via self-identification to Student Services or tutors.

- Include a question to identify young adult carers on enrolment form/online enrolment.
- Provide information about support for young adult carers at open days, in Student Services reception areas and in Student Union.
- Post intranet messages at the start of and throughout the year to encourage young adult carers to self-identify to Student Services.

If appropriate, initiate safeguarding.

Phase 2: Establish involvement of staff and other professionals

For example:

- University lead/champion for student carers.
- Personal tutor.
- Student mentor/representatives.
- Student Union.
- Student advisers.

Phase 3: Initiate university support systems

- Flexible learning and support.
- Personalised plan.
- Coursework/exam support.
- Peer support group.
- Young adult carers society.
- Staff to talk to/counselling.
- Emergency or crisis plan.
- Career advice service to support transition after university.

Phase 4: Initiate wider support from local services

To support the student:

- Use a multi-agency joint approach, for example with a young adult carers service, adult carers service, counselling service. Carers services will be able to support with assessing the student's needs in relation to their caring and if necessary, initiating support for their family.

To support the student's family: (better support for the student's family will help the student)

- Help student to access support for their family:
  - Adult social care.
  - Health services.
  - Carers services.
- Support student to request an assessment of their needs as a carer from their local authority. (An assessment should look at the needs of the whole family including any siblings who are caring).

Phase 5: Ensure ongoing monitoring

Student and family situations may change rapidly. Ongoing formal and informal monitoring is therefore important.

Source: Adapted from Carers Trust (2015).

Fig. 4.1. A Model for Working with Student Carers.

Carers' Employment Rights

Since the introduction of the Work and Families Act, 2006, employed carers have had the right to request flexible working from their employer. This right was extended as part of the Children and Families Act, 2014, to include carers' right to 'reasonable time off' if the person for whom they care is ill, injured or their care arrangements are disrupted.

The Equality Act, 2010, protects employees who are carers of 'a disabled or elderly person' from 'being treated less favourably' because of their association with someone who has a 'protected characteristic'.[6] This Act also protects them from discrimination by their employer, such as being treated 'less favourably' than others, for example, someone who is a not a carer.

The Carers Action Plan (2018–2020) sets out a number of actions to improve support for working carers. These include promoting best practice around flexible working and increasing opportunities for carers to return to work after caring has ended, in both the public and private sectors. There have also been consultations on proposals to introduce Carer's Leave: a right to 'one week's additional leave' for working carers. The Carer's Leave Act became law in May 2023 and will be enacted in 2024 (https://www.gov.uk/govern ment/news/boost-for-carers-who-will-receive-new-unpaid-lea ve-entitlement-under-government-backed-law) (Carers Trust, 2015; Fernandez et al., 2019; Powell et al., 2020).

In addition to these six broad areas of support for carers, temporary measures were introduced during the COVID pandemic across all four jurisdictions of the UK. In England entitlement to Carer's Allowance was continued during breaks in care if the carer, or the disabled person, had COVID or was self-isolating. In addition, providing 'emotional support' – including support provided remotely via the telephone or

---

6 Under the Equality Act 2010, there are nine protected characteristics: age, disability, gender reassignment, marriage and civil partnership, pregnancy and maternity, race, religion or belief, and sex. Having a protected characteristic means you have a right not to be treated less favourably, or subjected to an unfair disadvantage, by reason of that characteristic.

online – was included in the '35 hours a week of care' required to be eligible for Carer's Allowance. The Scottish Government issued advice for carers, including information on testing, and made a double payment of Carer's Allowance in June 2020 and December 2021. Guidance about infection control and sources of support was also issued for adult and young carers in Northern Ireland. The Welsh Government provided funding for services to help carers cope, e.g. online mental well-being support sessions (Foley et al., 2022).

The 2022 Health and Care Act aims to make carers a more visible partner in the health arena, engaging them in helping to shape services for their relatives and accord them additional rights. Specific provisions include: that carers must be involved 'as soon as possible' when plans for the patient's discharge from hospital are being made; a requirement that NHS Trusts involve carers in relation to any services for 'the prevention, diagnosis, care, and treatment of the person for whom they care'; and a duty that the NHS and Integrated Care Boards include carers in public consultations about care and support services and related policy and plans. Whilst these are all welcome aims, operationalising the development of a co-productive and inclusive approach to the design and delivery of care and support services is a challenge, particularly in the current financial climate (Kings Fund, 2022; Local Government Association, 2022).

OUTCOMES OF CARER-RELATED POLICES

Whilst carer-related policy in the UK is internationally recognised and emulated by other countries, for example Australia, there is a significant distance between the policy rhetoric and the realities of carers' lives. Of particular concern are reports that increasing numbers of people with care and support needs are seeking support from formal services as a direct consequence of carer breakdown or illness (ADASS, 2022; Carers Trust, 2022).

In order to provide a more in-depth assessment of the impact of carer-related policy in the UK we will now summarise evidence relating to outcomes for carers within the six key areas.

Benefits for Carers

In Chapter 3 we discussed the low level of Carer's Allowance. It is evidently not achieving its primary purpose of 'providing a measure of income maintenance in situations where a person cannot work full-time because of their caring responsibilities'. Not only is it the lowest non-means income replacement tested welfare benefit in the UK, it is also taxable. Furthermore, unlike other benefit recipients, carers are *not* entitled to free prescriptions, eye and dental care or subsidised travel (Carers Trust, 2022).

There has been much criticism of the restrictive nature of the criteria used to qualify for Carer's Allowance (see Box 4.1). Recipients are not allowed to be in full-time education and must only work up to an earnings threshold of £132 pw (in 2022) after deductions. This disqualifies many carers. Another criticism is that increases in the National Minimum Wage (now the National Living Wage (NLW)) mean carers working the 16 hours a week required to qualify for Working Tax Credit[7] can find themselves earning more than the Carer's Allowance earnings threshold. Carers are, in effect, obliged to choose between: (1) caring and education, (2) continuing in paid work and giving up their Carer's Allowance or

---

7 A state benefit in the UK to boost the income of people who work and have a low income.

(3) reducing their working hours to stay within the earnings limit and lose their Working Tax Credit.[8]

Unsurprisingly perhaps, only around 30% of claimants meet the criteria for Carer's Allowance. Table 4.2 shows that in November 2021 there were 1.3 million claimants (69% of whom were women). Of these only 70% *actually* received a payment. Exclusion on the grounds of receipt of other benefits (known as the overlapping benefits rule) resulted in only 4% of pensioners qualifying for Carer's Allowance in 2021 (Carers Trust, 2022). Whilst those who have reached State Pension age can apply for Attendance Allowance, they will only qualify for this benefit if they need 'help to manage activities of daily living as a consequence of a physical disability, a mental disability or both' and have 'needed that help for at least 6 months' (unless they are terminally ill). There are two rates. In 2022 the lower rate was £61.65 per week (for help during the day or at night); the higher rate was £92.40 per week (if help is needed *both* during the day and at night or in the case of a terminal illness). Attendance Allowance is paid to the person who needs help as opposed to Carer's Allowance which is paid to the carer.

Local Authority Support

The Care Act, 2014, provided parity of esteem for carers with adults with care and support needs according them a statutory right to an assessment of need and to have 'all eligible needs' met by their local authority. It was expected to lead to a substantial increase in the numbers of carers seeking assessments

---

8 Working Tax Credit is money provided to boost the income of working people who are on a low income. It counts as income when working out your entitlement to most other means-tested benefits.

Table 4.2. Carer's Allowance Claimants, Great Britain, November 2021.

	Total Claimants	Of Whom:	
		Male	Female
All claimants	**1,307,931**	**404,892**	**903,040**
Of whom: payment status:			
Claimant receiving payment	921,318	249,311	672,010
No payment: entitlement only	386,611	155,580	231,026
Receiving payment as % of total claimants	*70%*	*62%*	*74%*
Over State Pension age: total	**307,927**	**130,277**	**177,649**
Of whom: payment status:			
Claimant receiving payment	11,165	3,262	7,899
No payment: entitlement only	296,762	127,015	169,750
Receiving payment as % of pension age total	*4%*	*3%*	*4%*

Source: Adapted from Foley et al. (2022).

and support. Estimates suggested that it would generate an additional 270,000 carer assessments in the first year after its introduction, rising to a steady-state increase of 360,000 assessments per year by 2017–2018. The policy intention was that carer assessments would, amongst other things, be a route to carers gaining access to essential support.

Neither carers' enhanced rights to an assessment nor improved access to support has been realised. There has been a steady decline in the number of carer assessments since 2009/2010. Despite the heightened statutory rights of carers post the Care Act, between 2014–2015 and 2015–2016 there was a 14%

reduction in the number of assessments completed followed by a further decline of 6% in 2016–2017 (Fernandez et al., 2019). The total number of carers receiving an assessment of need has declined by nearly 50,000 over the last seven years. In 2021 it was estimated that only 24% of carers received assessments, or reassessments, of need (Carers UK, 2021a). In 2022 carers were often waiting 6 months or more for an assessment. Even when carer assessments *do* take place they are not necessarily a route to accessing support. National patterns hide significant local variation. In 2021 a number of local authorities reported conducting *three times as many* assessments as had been undertaken in 2019–2020, whilst others reported *two-thirds fewer* over the same period (ADASS, 2021).

The unrealised Care Act ambitions for carers have been, primarily, attributed to welfare austerity; local authority finances are in a parlous state after over a decade of cuts. Carers are one of the main casualties: carer-related expenditure has been reduced by 35% since 2014. This has been compounded by the fact that the model of support carers often need for their relative has been reduced significantly over the last 10 years, accelerated by the pandemic. Staff intensive services such as respite care and day care are in ever shorter supply; even where they exist there are significant staff recruitment and retention issues.

The impact of delays in carers assessments and the inadequacy of the support offered following an assessment are illustrated in the case study Robinder and Priti. Another potential contributory factor in their story is the considerable variation between local authorities in terms of service provision; some areas have a far greater number and range of services than others. Ironically, the more deprived an area is, the fewer public services there are. This is called the 'inverse care law'; where there is greatest need there tends to be the lowest level of support available (Fernandez et al., 2019; Marczak et al., 2022; Willis & Lloyd, 2021).

It is instructive to remind ourselves of the socio-demographic context outlined in Chapter 2. There are increasing numbers of older and disabled people *and* growing numbers of family carers; there are also more carers providing intensive care to relatives with complex co-morbid conditions. In other words, the lack of 'supply' of assessments and services is not about reduced 'demand'; it reflects an actual shrinking of 'supply', and an insufficient supply of particular kinds of services too.

Case Study: Robinder and Priti

Robinder has Parkinson's disease which affects his physical functioning and cognitive abilities. He uses a wheelchair and requires assistance moving around. Priti – his wife of 45 years – has managed his care without support for five years. However, she is now in her early seventies and it has come to the point where she is exhausted and needs help. She waited for an assessment of need from her local authority for over 4 months during which time Robinder's condition had deteriorated rapidly. When she finally did receive an assessment, she did not feel her needs were fully considered. Whilst her 'willingness and ability' to provide care was considered, her need to have regular breaks from caring, and to have time to herself, was overlooked.

The outcome of the assessment was that a home care service was provided morning and evening. This was only partially effective as the unpredictable nature of
                                                        (Continued)

(Continued)

Robinder's illness meant it was impossible for Priti to specify exactly when she needed help. The support provided was also rather limited and was not sufficiently tailored to Priti's specific situation. She did not really get a break from caring at all. Six months after the assessment, Priti collapsed from exhaustion and was admitted to hospital for three days. Emergency care had to be arranged; Robinder was admitted temporarily to a care home.

The high level of eligibility criteria for accessing publicly funded care means that assessments and services have become increasingly concentrated on carers providing intensive levels of care. There has also been a move away from the direct provision of services to the provision of 'information and advice'.

COVID has also had a significant impact. A lot of local authority funded support for both carers and adults with care and support needs was withdrawn, or severely reduced, during the pandemic. For example: day-care services closed, support groups were no longer offered or moved online and there were drastic reductions in the provision of home care and respite care in care homes. Resources were diverted to critical frontline and emergency support. Many carers also requested that services were withdrawn because of the (perceived) risk of them, or their relative, contracting the virus from care workers. This resulted in an intensification of care tasks for carers; 81% of carers provided more care during the pandemic and many experienced 'more negative' outcomes (see Chapter 3). Some carers were very proactive in addressing the challenges they faced, for example making more use of technology, accessing online resources provided by carers organisations and using the flexibility afforded them by being able to work from home (Carers UK, 2022a). However, there is growing evidence that reduced local authority support exacerbated pre-existing inequalities, particularly in relation to (further) deterioration in carers' physical and mental health. Many services that closed during the pandemic have either not reopened post pandemic or have only opened on a part-time basis, due to ongoing resource constraints.

Of those carers who do gain access to formal support less than 40% say they are 'satisfied' with services; satisfaction rates are also falling. One cause of dissatisfaction is that the support does not meet their specific needs; services are insufficiently nuanced (see Case Study above). This is particularly the case if carers are from an ethnic minority, or an under-represented, community. Table 4.3 demonstrates how

Table 4.3. Carer's Satisfaction Rate with Support Services.

Ethnicity	
White British Carers	28%
Other White Background	35%
Asian/Asian British Carers	29%
Black/Black British Carers	32%
Carers from a Mixed/Multiple ethnic background	28%
Sexual orientation	
Heterosexual Carers	28%
Gay/Lesbian Carers	30%
Bisexual Carers	33%
Disability	
Non-disabled Carers	27%
Disabled Carers	33%

Source: Carers UK (2021a).

satisfaction levels vary according to carers' ethnicity, sexual orientation and whether or not they are disabled (Carers UK, 2021a; NHS Digital, 2019). Services have also been criticised for being unreliable and/or inadequate. Common complaints include: poor quality 'replacement care' resulting in carers and their relatives refusing to consider it again; flying visits from home care workers who barely have the time to complete basic tasks and workers routinely being late and/or poorly trained (Carers Trust, 2022).

Given the profile of lack of access to assessments or support, it is not surprising that in a recent survey only 7% of carers said they received 'sufficient support' and just 13% reported that they were 'confident that they were going to get the support they needed in the next 12 months' (Carers Trust, 2022). The Care Act's aim to ensure carers gain access to effective support appears less likely than ever to be realised (Carers UK, 2021a; Cheshire-Allen & Calder, 2022; Cipolletta et al., 2021).

The fact that many carers, and cared-for people, are simply not getting the support that they need not only threatens carer quality of life and increases the risk of carer breakdown but it (often) means that working carers are obliged to choose between paid work and care (see Chapter 3). It is widely known that giving up work prematurely increases the risk of poverty. This trend – made worse by COVID – has prompted fears that poverty will affect more families with dependent members. The cost-of-living crisis deepens these fears (ADASS, 2021, 2022; Carers UK, 2022b). There are also growing concerns that expectations we will all need to work for longer will (further) erode opportunities for employed carers to 'retire early' or reduce working hours to provide care.

Carer Health and Well-Being

The absence of progress on improving carer health and well-being is reflected in the continuation of high rates of physical and psychological ill-health amongst carers outlined in Chapter 3. Not only is this failure to deliver improved outcomes for carers a matter of social justice, but it is an essential component of sustainable care (Keating et al., 2021). These are issues to which we return in later chapters.

Young Carers

Studies show that fewer than one in five young carers receive an assessment of their needs and nearly two-thirds (64%) receive *no support* from any source. Of those receiving help, the most common source is a young carers' project, e.g. a summer holiday programme, followed by support via their school or college such as a young carers group or counselling. Although direct support to young carers via their school has been found to be very effective, research suggests that only about 1 in 10 young carers gain access to this kind of help (Foley et al., 2022).

Despite the fact that Carer's Allowance can be claimed from the age of 16, the eligibility criteria mean that any young carer in full-time education is excluded from claiming (as noted above). The rationale is that people in full-time education, including those with caring responsibilities, are already supported through the educational maintenance system via its portfolio of loans and grants. However, critics argue, it is very likely that many young carers miss out on support, being excluded from claiming Carer's Allowance *and* from benefitting from the educational maintenance system.

At present, families with young carers may get additional help through the Severe Disability Premium (SDP), worth £69.40 a week (2022/2023 rate). SDP is intended to give 'additional help to severely disabled people'. It is not a benefit as such but an additional amount payable with certain means-tested benefits. However, benefit changes taking place between 2022 and 2026 – involving the replacement of existing means-tested benefits and tax credits for working-age families by Universal Credit (UC) – will mean there will be *no* equivalent to the SDP. There are concerns this could have a disproportionate impact on poverty rates amongst families with young carers, thereby increasing the poverty-related disadvantages they are exposed to (Cheesbrough et al., 2017; Foley et al., 2022).

The importance of helping young carers to participate 'more fully in social and educational life' and prevent damage to their long-term educational and health outcomes is well documented (Cheesbrough et al., 2017). Evidence about the high proportion of young carers who do not access support underscores the need for more to be done. There are a number of ways forward. One suggestion is around developing new, and strengthening existing, relationships between young carers' services and schools with the aims of: maximising the adoption of sustainable, 'whole school approaches' to identifying and supporting young carers; and encouraging schools to proactively build, or maintain, links with their local young carers service (Carter, 2017). Other ways forward include targeted work with more marginalised groups of young carers via outreach workers (e.g. in BAME communities) and ensuring that health and social care agencies communicate information about the availability and nature of young carers' services more effectively (Jacklin, 2021; James, 2019). Often overlooked in policymaking is addressing the obstacles to recognition and identification of young carers because they fear stigmatisation and bullying. Families also fear disclosure because of potential 'repercussions' such as the adult with care and support needs being 'removed' or the young carer being taken into the care of the local authority (Cheesbrough et al., 2017; Foley et al., 2022). These are difficult barriers to tackle.

Carers and Higher Education

Whilst the inclusion of carers under the umbrella of widening participation in higher education is to be welcomed, studies show that student carers often experience considerable challenges balancing their commitments to study, provide care and (often) do paid work. As a consequence of these difficulties, the attrition rate for student carers is four times higher than it is for other students (Kettell, 2020).

Despite their raised profile, there is very limited knowledge about the needs of student carers and how best to support them. College and University strategies are underdeveloped (Larkin & Kubiak, 2021). There have been calls for further research and regular sharing of good practice in this area; also the development of higher education-wide plans to support student carers and improve their engagement with, and retention within, higher education. Specific suggestions include: providing financial aid (e.g. carer bursaries) and advice; establishing systems to identify student carers; building more flexibility into curriculum design (e.g. study breaks) and social engagement opportunities that student carers can fit in around their commitments (e.g. online peer support groups) (Larkin & Kubiak, 2021; Overgaard & Mackaway, 2022).

Growing care demands are likely to be reflected in an increase in the number of students with caring responsibilities. There is clearly a need for a targeted and multifaceted approach to identifying and supporting student carers if they are to be retained in higher education and to realise academic opportunities.

Carers' Employment Rights

Considerable progress has been made in relation to carers' employment rights. There is now much greater recognition of the valuable role carers play in the workplace. Many organisations across the public, private and voluntary sectors have introduced carer-friendly employment policies as a result of legislation, campaigning and raised public awareness. A key example of this is reflected in the growth in membership of Employers for Carers. As can be seen from Box 4.4, this is an organisation which supports employers in managing and retaining employees with caring responsibilities.

Box 4.4

· ·

Employers for Carers

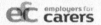

Launched in 2009 Employers for Carers (EfC) has evolved from a pioneering group of organisations committed to working carers to a multi-sector forum, supported by the specialist knowledge of Carers UK.

EfC now has over 245 member organisations across the public, private and voluntary sectors, covering over 3.8 million employees. Their purpose is to ensure that employers have the support to retain and empower employees with caring responsibilities. Through its

---

(*Continued*)

innovative platform *Employers for Carers Digital*, consultancy and support programmes help employers to identify the needs of staff with caring responsibilities and promote effective workplace practices to support them and their managers. There is evidence that those employers reap the business benefits of doing so in terms of better engaged staff, lower recruitment costs and turnover, and retention of talent and experience.

Source: *EFC (employersforcarers.org)*.

Evaluations of employers' carer-related policies suggest that the following flexibilities are effective ways to promote working carer well-being and retention: being permitted to take private calls associated with caring during the working day; flexible work arrangements (including working from home) and taking unpaid leave to deal with care-related crises and demands (Austin & Heyes, 2020; Wilson et al., 2018). One of the weaknesses of the current model is that it requires individual workers to self-identify as carers. Much depends on the attitude of their line manager; s/he may, or may not, be sympathetic and may, or may not, consider a request for 'flexible working' or 'unpaid leave'. What is clear is that much more needs to be done by way of workplace support to reduce the number of carers who are obliged to either work fewer hours or give up work altogether due to their caring responsibilities. The government's commitment to introducing carers leave and making flexible working the 'default position' have yet to be adopted widely by employers; the 2023 Carer's Leave Act is likely to make some positive difference to employed carers (Foley et al., 2022; Williams & Bank, 2022; Wilson et al., 2018).

As noted above, the pandemic meant that many carers found themselves navigating additional care responsibilities without the usual levels of support from family, friends or services. Although being able to work from home gave (some) carers more flexibility in carrying out their caring tasks, the lack of boundary between work and home can be damaging to carer well-being. Adapting to different ways of working and taking on more care tasks with depleted resources generated considerable stress for many carers and, as discussed in Chapter 3, elevated their anxiety and stress levels (Lafferty et al., 2022).

The 'personalisation agenda' also has implications for carers. Personalisation emphasises the role of direct payments[9], as a mechanism for enabling (eligible) service users to determine their own care priorities. There is evidence that carers are often obliged to spend time on the administrative responsibilities involved in managing a direct payment, such as organising care services or employing a personal assistant. Carers sometimes refer to themselves as 'care managers'. Whilst some carers experience this role as beneficial in terms of facilitating greater levels of choice, others report being anxious about the planning and management of their relative's care package – anxieties which are compounded by the lack of diversity and availability in the local care market. They also worry about money and following all the administrative procedures 'correctly' (Larkin & Mitchell, 2016).

In sum, two things stand out from our analysis. It is clear that policy-related achievements are relatively modest in scale and

---

9 Direct payments are cash payments made to individuals assessed by their local authority as being eligible to receive services. They are in lieu of local authority organised provision. The person uses the payment to purchase their own care and support.

ambition. Also, they tend to be opaque; where a concrete service or benefit does exist, it is a challenge to access and retain.

SUPPORT FOR CARER POPULATIONS

Inequalities in accessing services have been amplified by the COVID pandemic. Some of the inequalities in the support different groups of carers receive were explored in Sections 1 and 2 – namely young carers and working carers. We are now going to take a closer look at how access to support, and outcomes, vary for some of the other groups of carers explored in Chapters 2 and 3.

BAME Carers

Research shows that BAME carers are less likely to receive 'practical and financial support' and more likely to miss out on accessing 'all services' than other groups of carers. This has been attributed, in part at least, to the lack of advice and information in appropriate languages and also few culturally appropriate services. That asking for help is often viewed as stigmatising because the term 'carer' is counter-cultural and conflicts with notions of 'duty to care' for relatives is also relevant. Particular conditions, such as HIV, mental illness, dementia and learning disabilities, can be a source of stigma for some cultures too, e.g. the Asian cultures (Carers UK, 2019a; Nair et al., 2022).

Sandwich Carers

Sandwich carers may be able to access some support, e.g. benefits. If they are working, they may also have access to employment-related carer support. Studies show that sandwich carers are more likely to struggle financially and with their mental health too. Despite campaigns there is a lack of targeted support for this group of carers (Oldridge & Larkin, 2020; Embracing Carers, 2021).

Older Carers

Older carers routinely report feeling unsupported. This has been linked to a number of factors. As discussed in Chapter 2, many older carers, especially spouses, are hidden from view and tend not to identify as a carer. Older carers are often reluctant to ask for help and tend to resist the 'intrusion' of outsiders (including services). Even when they do seek support, there can be a lack of 'fit' between older carers' needs and service models. One of the main reasons is that services tend to focus on instrumental care tasks such as helping with bathing rather than supporting the intensive emotional work often associated with caring in later life, such as bolstering the cared-for person's role and identity. The cared-for person may also be unwilling to accept input from services (Embracing Carers, 2021; Larkin et al., 2020).

The way that the overlapping benefits rule works means that only 4% of pensioners qualify for Carer's Allowance (referred to above). Although this fact continues to cause confusion, anger and distress amongst older carers, successive governments have resisted calls to abolish this rule (Powell et al., 2020).

Dementia Carers

Despite the fact that caring for a person living with dementia is one of the most challenging caring roles, many dementia carers care unaided. As a high proportion of dementia carers are older spouses, they share a number of the features noted above, for example, resisting self-identifying and not accepting help from relatives or services. The person living with dementia may also be unwilling to acknowledge there is 'anything wrong with them'. Those dementia carers with the greatest capacity to cope tend to be embedded in contexts where they have strong family support, a healthy financial situation, input from formal services and/or the person they care for is in the early stages of the condition with few symptoms (Oliveira et al., 2019).

One of the long-standing criticisms of the way people living with dementia and their carers are supported is to assess, and support, them separately. There is a call for the care system to recognise that (most) dementia caring takes place within the context of a dyadic relationship. Assessment and the planning of care and support should therefore be based on the adoption of a dyadic lens. The fact that a service for one member of the dyad may have a positive impact on the other, e.g. day care, underscores this need (Quinn et al., 2022; Rand et al., 2022).

Former Carers

Although former carers are beginning to have a more visible public profile, there is very limited formal support for this group of carers. One of the main reasons for this is that once carers are no longer 'actively' caring, they are not regarded by statutory agencies as justifying assessments of need or access to support. If a carer had joined a carer support group earlier in their care trajectory, they tend to continue to attend it post caring. Some third sector carers organisations even offer specific support groups to former carers. Bereaved former carers may also access bereavement counselling or support groups from specialist bereavement services (Larkin & Milne, 2017, 2021).

Family Members Supporting a Relative With a Terminal Illness

National palliative and end-of-life services now promote comprehensive, holistic carer assessment and support and a person-centred approach for carers as well as patients. This reflects the growing recognition of the central role that family carers play in supporting relatives with a terminal illness (Carers Trust, 2019; Ewing & Grande, 2018).

This review of evidence makes it clear that support for carers is underfunded, fragmented, limited and varies according to where the carer lives and what happens to be available locally. Deficits in the provision of support impact negatively on the health and well-being of carers and undermines their ability to care in the way they would wish. Research consistently highlights the lack of pro-active practical support and inconsistency in the quality and availability of services. Communication about the nature of support is an issue too, for example, family carers often do not know who is coming to their home, how often and at what times. Gaps in support are also linked to the welfare of family carers themselves. Carers routinely report that their own needs are overlooked and identify the following as particular deficits: respite care, nuanced individualised assessments of need, counselling and assessment of carers' own health conditions (Ateş et al., 2018; Morris et al., 2015).

CARER SUPPORT AND POLICY: SOME REFLECTIONS

One of the primary aims of all carer-related policies and strategies is to provide more, and more effective, support for carers. At present, there is limited evidence that this is translated into practice in any meaningful or sustained way. Even when carers do receive support, it is not necessarily effective. Central to debates about carer-related policy are a number of long-standing challenges. Arguably the most important is funding. Supporting carers adequately costs money; however good a policy is, if it is not supported by public funding, its wings will be clipped. This is certainly the case for the Care Act, 2014.

Another challenge relates to carer identification. As noted above, many carers do not self-identify and professionals do not routinely identify carers either. Any policy predicated on carers owning the label of 'carer' will fall at the first hurdle if those doing the caring remain hidden. Whilst this reflects, to some degree, the ambiguous relationship carers have with policy and services, i.e. we rely on carers to do caring with minimal input from the state, there are other factors at play too. One of these is the complex interaction between 'support' and 'effectiveness'. Effectiveness has been found to be shaped by (at least) the following dimensions: heterogeneity of care situations; different care trajectories; and the stage of caring. These are, in turn, shaped by: the characteristics of the care recipients; the nature of the care relationship; the effect of unmet needs; social networks; technological innovations (e.g. to improve carers, manage conditions and access services); and culture and inequalities including gender, age, socio-economic status, race and sexuality (Cartagena-Farias & Brimblecombe, 2022; Fast et al., 2021; Nolan et al., 1996).

One of the reasons we struggle with the concept of 'effective support' is that it means different things to different groups of carers *and* individuals. It is not surprising that most research on 'effectiveness' tends to be done on a specific group of carers, e.g. older carers, around a particular condition, e.g. dementia, or on a specific intervention or service. Capturing effectiveness more widely is almost impossible; there are simply too many factors to accommodate. Evidence is strongest in relationship to interventions for groups of carers, such as carers of people with dementia, cancer or stroke. There are huge gaps in existing research; the research that does exist on effectiveness is of mixed quality (Brimblecombe et al., 2018b; Larkin et al., 2019).

Suggestions have been made about the future direction of research on services and service effectiveness. For example, there have been calls for more good quality, theory-based, primary research which adopts a lens of analysis that captures what carers say would help them across their whole care trajectory (Cipolletta et al., 2021; Dalton et al., 2018). This 'caring life course' lens would accommodate the notion of effectiveness on a temporal, more flexible and nuanced basis than current 'snapshot' approaches to research do. Others have identified the need for systemic changes in terms of improving access to the health and social care system. A key proposal relates to ensuring carers have access to a trusted knowledgeable professional who: recognises their concerns, challenges, needs and rights; provides tailored advice about services and benefits; and can help them navigate the care system (Butt, 2020; Embracing Carers, 2021). Another idea relates to personal finances; it has been suggested that financial advisors could explore their client's current and future care responsibilities when developing and revising financial plans (Duncan et al., 2020).

CONCLUDING COMMENTS

Supporting carers is everyone's business and, yet somehow, it is nobody's. Caring intersects with many different policy agendas and interleaves with most aspects of daily life. It is not just about health and social care but also public, private and voluntary organisations and also employers and the benefits system. These all need to adapt and change in order to support the growing and increasingly heterogeneous population(s) of carers. There is a particular challenge to reduce the inequalities experienced by carers generally and by specific groups of carers in particular.

Such transformational change needs strong leadership from government. It requires political will. That the UK government – and the policy infrastructure – can deliver transformational change at pace was witnessed during the COVID pandemic. The furlough scheme and the mass vaccination programme are examples of this. Carers organisations have been campaigning for this level, and range, of response to be applied to meeting the needs of carers for many years (Carers Trust, 2022). How we understand and conceptualise family care informs the socio-political agenda and policy responses to carers. It permeates the language used to describe 'care' in public discourse and who 'qualifies' for carer-related support. It is pivotal to the care debate and it is to this issue that we turn in Chapter 5.

5

CONCEPTUALISING AND UNDERSTANDING CARE AND CARING

INTRODUCTION

Both Chapters 5 and 6 build on the evidence presented in Chapters 2–4 about the profile of carers, what they do, the impact of caring on carers' lives and health, and policy and support for carers.

The aim of Chapter 5 is to add a conceptual and theoretical dimension to the carer-related discussion. It is important work because it helps to widen our understanding of care and the complexities associated with caring (Ray et al., 2009). It also locates care firmly inside the research arena and makes its links to policy and the political sphere more visible. We acknowledge that the tone of this chapter, and Chapter 6, is inevitably more academic and analytical than earlier chapters as the material being reviewed demands it, but we have tried to make it as accessible as possible. There is a greater intersection between the process of caring, care and carers too. Where appropriate, links are made with earlier chapters and examples given.

The chapter is made up of two main sections: 'Conceptualising Care: Approaches and Lenses' and 'Understanding the Nature of Care and Caring'. These outline different per-spectives on the concepts – and meanings – of care, carer and caring and how they intersect and engage with the ways that we think about family care. What influences our understanding is explored and challenges to traditional assumptions about care are made.

We begin with a brief overview of key issues.

Although family carers have always existed, the term 'carer' was not formally recognised in the UK until the early 1980s and in many languages and countries it remains unac-knowledged as a role. It was only in the latter 20 years of the twentieth century that caring was identified as an issue for social policy and services and that carers became the focus of empirical and academic research (Barnes, 2006). As noted in Chapter 2, although the word carer is widely accepted in public and policy discourse, it remains a contested term (Larkin & Milne, 2014). Its hidden private nature contributes to its off-the-radar status; that care is viewed by some as a normal part of a familial role contributes to its invisibility.

Caring incorporates a number of dimensions: it involves tasks, roles and relationships. It can be situated along a number of intersecting axes. Early feminist writers observed that caring is both about love and about labour; carers care *about* the person they support and simultaneously care *for* them (Graham, 1991). This work not only highlighted the gendered nature of (most) family care but also its multidi-mensionality. The fact that caring is routinely constructed as 'natural' for women underpins what Sevenhuijsen (1998) terms the 'silent logic' of its persistently gendered profile (Hughes et al., 2005). Care is often embedded in a long-term relationship such as marriage, but it is also about the delivery of care tasks. Care incorporates the instrumental (e.g. help-ing someone to eat), physical (e.g. helping them to get upstairs), the emotional, the social and the practical (e.g.

washing soiled bed linen) (Finch & Groves, 1983). Caring is often emotionally complex, engendering a mixture of feelings: love, guilt, anger, resentment, compassion and pity.

Care is also delivered in the moment but may be the product of a lifetime of interactions and commitments (Yeandle et al., 2017). Reciprocity, i.e. the mutual exchange of help and support, is often a key dimension of care. Most carers feel obliged to care, even if they do so willingly, and cannot be assumed to put their needs above those of the cared-for person (as noted in earlier chapters). This is a particular risk if they do not define themselves as a carer. Care is always a product of, and is situated in, a relational and social context. This is one of the reasons it is such a challenge to define and capture as it takes myriad forms and shapes, is dynamic and shifts through time, across cultures and the life course (Phillips, 2007). Whilst some caring experiences are shared by most carers, e.g. feeling trapped, other elements are more particular to specific circumstances, contexts or life stages. A parent caring for a physically disabled child, for example, is a very different experience from a mid-life daughter caring for her frail elderly mother. Similarly, a younger spouse supporting their partner with multiple sclerosis is likely to be facing (some) very different challenges to an older spouse caring for a partner with dementia.

A fundamental contradiction also underpins family care: it is vital to human flourishing but is often taken for granted, treated as ordinary and not worthy of attention (Yeandle et al., 2017). Family care is 'the oft overlooked scaffolding of our lives, on which well-being and daily life depend' (Bunting, 2016, p. 33). Care, caring and carer are simultaneously complex and seductively simple terms.

CONCEPTUALISING CARE: APPROACHES
AND LENSES

Care and caring are the subject of a number of different, but interconnected, conceptual and analytical lenses (Phillips, 2007). Although there is now a rich literature on care and caring, it is important to acknowledge it is 'work in progress'. The field is characterised by a number of key building blocks of material drawn from a number of different academic and research related sources. Whilst space does not permit a review of the whole field – it is huge – we offer a synthesis of the core dimensions of the discourse, the key lenses adopted, and main approaches taken to understanding and exploring care and caring. Whilst a number of these issues have been raised in earlier chapters, here they are drawn together in a single narrative. As will be obvious to the reader by now, the care arena is characterised by features that interleave in multiple ways.

Where a specific group of carers, e.g. dementia carers, make visible a particular set of conceptual issues these are highlighted.

CARING AS A TEMPORAL JOURNEY

As identified in Chapter 3, a significant contribution to understanding caring has been made by work exploring the care journey and the roles that carers (often) adopt relating to that journey. The most long-standing models conceptualise caring as existing on a continuum from pre-caring through to post-caring; it is sometimes termed a caregiving trajectory.

Seminal foundational work – upon which others have built – was done in the mid-1990s. For example, Nolan et al. (1996) developed a typology of care drawing on work by

Bowers (1987, 1988). Their model identifies 6 stages of care: anticipatory care; preventive care; supervisory care; instrumental care; protective/preservative care and reconstructive care (See Table 5.1: examples of care activity that relates to each stage of care is identified in the third column).

Table 5.1. Typology of Care.

Stage of Care	Meaning of Stage	Example of Activity
Anticipatory care	Preparing for future caring responsibilities	An older couple one of whom has dementia may move closer to their daughter
Preventive care	Monitoring at a distance	Keeping an eye on medication management
Supervisory care	Actively engaging with activities	Making sure medication is taken, enough food is eaten and showers are regularly taken
Instrumental care	Doing physical and/or personal care tasks	Helping with dressing, bathing, personal care
Protective/ preservative care	Preserving as much of the cared-for person's functioning as possible	Ensuring their daily routines are maintained and all existing functions are promoted
Reconstructive care (post admission to care home)	Developing a new role(s)	Informing the care staff about the life history and character of the cared-for person (especially important if they have dementia)

Source: Adapted from Nolan et al. (1996).

Anticipatory care is described as 'just in case' and is about relatives preparing for likely future caring responsibilities. It is more commonly experienced by adult children in relationship to their parents; also spouses to some degree. It tends to persist as a 'type' of care throughout the whole caring journey. The main component of preventive care is 'monitoring at a distance'. It shares this feature with anticipatory care but is more active. For example, it may involve a carer keeping an eye on medication usage and supplies, that the person's eating habits are healthy, and they are drinking enough water. When such a monitoring role requires more direct intervention, such as actual assistance with taking medication, then supervisory care may be required. Instrumental care involves helping with mobility, e.g. getting up and downstairs, and personal care, e.g. bathing and washing; it may also involve help with feeding.

Protective, preservative and reconstructive care are interlinked. Bowers (1987, 1988) conceptualised protective care as being primarily concerned with keeping the cared-for person 'protected' from being made aware of their reduced abilities and increasing dependency. She later substituted the concept of preservative care, the purpose being to maintain as much of the person's functioning as possible. The purpose of (re) constructive care is to 'build upon the past' in order to develop new roles. This type of care intersects with preservative care, particularly in contexts where the cared-for person has a deteriorating condition such as dementia.

Nolan et al. (1996) regard reciprocal care as an overarching concept which underpins and informs the typology; it wraps around the whole notion of family care. Whilst this may be challenging in contexts of chronic or progressive decline such as dementia, in most care relationships reciprocity is the foundation of care before, during – and for some – after the period of care has ended. For example, in contexts where the cared-for person recovers from an illness, such as cancer. Whilst direct exchanges of instrumental care are unlikely in the later stages of most care relationships, this ignores the myriad ways in which reciprocity operates. It may be psychological, material, financial; it may also be diffuse and subtle and is often linked to lifelong exchanges, not necessarily exchanges in the recent past. A daughter's commitment to her mother is (often) based on what her mother did for her earlier in life not what her mother offered her in the last few years. The roots of reciprocity are long and they run deep. Reciprocity is also a core dimension of the ethic of care approach discussed in the next section.

Nolan et al.'s (1996) conceptual model is partly rooted in sequential stages of caregiving and partly not. It acknowledges that some care roles take shape later in the development of a condition but, at the same time, recognises that other roles exist throughout the whole care trajectory and may take a different form as the trajectory unfolds. Anticipatory care, for example, does not disappear when instrumental care becomes needed. At an earlier stage the carer may anticipate needing to help their relative manage a task such as responding to e-mails but later on they may anticipate needing to arrange input from formal care services such as home care. More 'types' of care tend to be required over time; care demands tend to increase and multiply. Intensive carers – carers who tend to do many hours of care and tasks that are more demanding such as bathing and dressing – also need to manage less intensive types of care, such as arranging hospital appointments and ordering medication (see Chapter 2). These issues speak to the incremental and increasing demands of caregiving over time as well as its complex and dynamic nature.

Although other more recent models build on this early work, the nature of the caregiving journey and the identified stages remain a consistent feature. Terminology may vary, for example, 'expectant carer' in place of 'anticipatory care' but the role is the same. More recent work places greater emphasis on the caring experience as an emotional journey as well as a practical one. This is an issue to which we return later in the chapter.

Subsequent work by Davies and Nolan (2004, 2006), and others, recognised that the carer's role may extend beyond the admission of a – usually older – relative to a care home. Three additional phases were added to the model. The first two – the 'decision-making process' and making arrangements for 'moving into the care home' – occur pre-admission. The third phase – 'making it better' – occurs post-admission and involves the carer establishing a new 'carer role'. The carer role often includes helping with mealtimes and/or bathing their relative; it may also involve ensuring that the care staff know about the person's character, history, tastes and likes/dislikes, e.g. about food or TV programmes (Larkin & Milne, 2021).

Larkin's (2009) work developed the concept of a distinctive post-caring trajectory comprising three phases. The first two are the 'post-caring void' and 'closing down the caring time' whilst the third – 'constructing life post-caring' – involves getting 'life together' again, during which former carers reconnect with their families, pursue their interests and take up new activities. Cronin et al. (2015) conceptualise the post-caring period as a time of being 'between worlds' during which former carers experience three iterative inter-related transitions: 'loss of the caring world', 'living in loss' and 'moving on'. This work shares some conceptual terrain with work on end-of-life and palliative carers discussed below.

CARING ROLE AND CARER IDENTITY

There is a developing body of work, drawn mainly from the field of psychology, on the adoption of the carer role and the development of a carer identity.

Social identity theory (Tajfel & Turner, 1979) suggests that individuals have a repertoire of social and personal identities the importance of which vary over time. As already noted, the onset of chronic illness, and deterioration in health of a spouse, makes new demands on their partner. Over time they are likely to become increasingly involved in caring activities and may well experience a loss of identity as a partner and companion (Henderson, 2001). Other personal and social identities may also be lost; a carer may be obliged to give up their hobbies and interests such as membership of a reading group or volunteering at a foodbank. This change is not only about the loss of roles in the present but the loss of anticipated activities and plans for the future. Bury's (1982) work on biographical disruption describes chronic illness as a 'fundamental rupture in the fabric of everyday life', and a resulting disruption of the narratives about the future that people use to understand themselves and the trajectories of their lives (p. 167). Meeting the challenge of caring over time may involve significant biographical adjustment on the part of a carer (See section on 'Dementia Care' below).

Drawing on social identity theory, Montgomery and Kosloski (2013) developed a specific 'theory of caregiver identity'. It is based on three premises, that: the caring role is acquired in a systematic way, it is a dynamic process that changes over time and as carers' experience a change in their role, they also experience a change in their identity. This theory identifies common elements of the caring role whilst acknowledging that, for each individual, the role is acquired and experienced differently depending on the nature of the care relationship, cultural and familial experiences, societal expectations and structural assumptions, e.g. about gender roles. At its most fundamental level, the caring experience is characterised by two factors: the activities in which the carer is engaging and the meaning that s/he attaches to these (Skaff & Pearlin, 1992). This seemingly obvious observation has profound implications for the study of caring. First, it means that caring is not a 'unitary process'; the process will be different for each disease trajectory and each relationship. Second, it means that the same caring activities can be perceived differently, depending upon a range of factors that influence the caring context, e.g. income, support from other family members. It is '… the totality of these factors, that define each caregiving experience and uniquely identify caregivers one from another' (Montgomery & Kosloski, 2013, p. 136).

Carer identity is also affected by the quantity and intensity of the needs of the cared-for person. As noted in earlier chapters, this shifts over time. The initial (usually) familial relationship 'gives way to a relationship characterised by caregiving' (Montgomery & Kosloski, 2013, p. 137). Caring activities can transform the original relationship – for example, mother–daughter – into a caring relationship. When caring demands can be easily assimilated into the carer's existing identity as daughter minimal distress is experienced, but as the discrepancy between the caring activities and her self-identity increases, psychological distress increases too (Stryker & Burke, 2000). For example, the daughter may decide that in order to manage her discomfort in helping to bathe her mother she needs to accept that she is now her mother's carer and identify as such, reflecting a change in their mother–daughter relationship. If she has the resources she may, on the other hand, employ a care worker to bathe her mother, thereby retaining her identity as a daughter. She may also arrange to regularly have coffee with her mother – a routine they may have had for many years – to reinforce the original mother–daughter relationship.

Montgomery and Kosloski (2013) argue that carer-related stress is the product of at least one of the following: a discrepancy between the way the carer views herself relative to her caring activities; a change in the way in which she views the relationship with her relative; and/or a fundamental change in the caring situation, e.g. a significant deterioration in the cared-for person's health. Each of these factors has different implications for the need for, and ultimately the efficacy of, a support service. The theory of caregiver identity is advanced as a framework to help service providers under-stand the sources of carer stress, effectively target support and aid policymakers to design support systems that meet carers' needs. It draws on an individual microperspective on stress complementing the broader contextual and sociostructural causes of stress discussed in Chapter 3.

The theory of caregiver identity also intersects with seminal work by Lewis and Meredith in the late 1980s/1990s (1989). They explored the extent to which caring is integrated into a carer's life, identifying three broad categories. These are: the 'balanced mode' in which carers are able to combine caring with other key roles in their lives such as paid employment; the 'integrated mode' where caring provides a sense of pur-pose, identity and satisfaction for the carer; and the 'immersed carer' who invests heavily in caring and finds it extremely difficult to accommodate any other role in their life or to move on when caring comes to an end. For example, a long-term carer may struggle to adapt to a new life after caring ends. It is no coincidence that many of those who volunteer to work in carers' third sector agencies are ex-carers themselves (Larkin, 2009). It is a role they know well and feel confident about advising on. This conceptualisation has resonance with Twigg and Atkin's (1994) carer typology, discussed later in this Chapter.

DEMENTIA CARE

Due to its complexity as a condition, the (often) long trajectory of care and the range and types of challenges carers often face, dementia care has been the focus of specific research attention (Nolan et al., 2001, 2003). In the dementia arena, caring is more clearly embedded in sequential iterative stages. Although the speed and precise nature of the care trajectory will differ by person, dyad and context for most dementia carers, caring becomes increasingly more intensive as the condition progresses. Dementia care is viewed as beginning pre-diagnosis and ending when the person with dementia dies.

An early model by Wilson (1989) identified eight stages: noticing, discounting/normalising, suspecting, searching for explanations, recounting (once a diagnosis is made, retrospective reappraisal of what has gone before), taking it on (assuming a care role and, for some, decisions about future care options), going through it (supporting an increasingly frail and dependent person); and turning it over (recognition that the carer's own physical and mental health is suffering and that other options may need to be considered).

Based on research with carers and people living with dementia, Keady and Nolan (1994, 2003) refined this and developed a six-stage model:

- Building on the past (appreciating the nature and quality of the past relationship)
- Recognising the need ('noticing')
- Taking on the caring role

- Working through it ('going through it')

- Reaching the end (the end of hands-on instrumental care, often accompanied by physical separation of the carer and cared-for person by care home admission)

- A new beginning (adjusting to a different life and for those whose relative is in a care home, a new type of caring role)

One of the main drivers for this work on dementia care models was to help inform when, and how, service-related interventions could dovetail most effectively with supporting carers. These models retain relevance to the current dementia care paradigm as the stages of dementia care are (largely) the same. What is different now is that there are many more people with dementia living in the community being supported by a family carer; dementia carers are also doing more complex and intensive care tasks for longer and with more limited (if any) support from services (as noted in Chapter 2–4).

Research on dementia care has delineated three 'types' of 'care work': physical labour, organisational/managerial labour and emotional labour (James, 1992). Physical labour is the most visible type of care work, helping the person with activities of daily living such as eating, bathing/washing, dressing/undressing and using the toilet. Some commentators distinguish between 'illness specific work' such as managing medication and 'everyday work' including personal care (Knowles et al., 2016). Managerial labour includes organising input from formal care services, ensuring 'cover' is available when the carer is doing paid work and/or ordering medications or aids. Emotional labour refers to the way in which people manage their emotions in order to protect the feelings of the person they are looking after (Hochschild, 2012). This may include hiding upset about loss of cognitive function or masking the negative impact of disturbed nights (Vassilev et al., 2013). It is a concept more usually applied to paid work and is discussed in relationship to care workers later in the chapter. Although physical labour is the most obvious form of caring, organisational labour and emotional labour are often needed first; they represent what has changed for the cared-for person and in the relationship. Although we are talking about dementia care in this section, these types of care work are also relevant to carers of people with other long-term conditions.

Another lens on dementia caring relates to loss and grief. Loss is a key feature of conceptual and applied work in this field. Dementia grief has been described as a specific type of anticipatory grief (Santulli & Blandin, 2015). Although anticipatory grief can occur in many terminal illnesses, dementia grief is distinguished by disruptions in communication and impairments of awareness that often accompany dementia. Many dementia carers are exposed to 'compounded serial losses'; these build in magnitude and number as the condition progresses. Early losses include memory and communication deficits; advanced losses include a decline in ability to dress or bathe and/or recognise the carer.

Dementia grief is characterised by 'ambiguous loss'. Ambiguous loss is experienced as 'a lack of clarity due to losses that are unstable and fluctuating evading resolution', for example the resolution of past marital conflicts (Blandin & Pepin, 2017, p. 70). Diminution of (some) identifying personality characteristics and the inability to access personal memories is also a feature of ambiguous loss. Sharing memories is one of the ways that older couples reinforce their marriage and identity as a couple (Hyden & Nilsson, 2015). Due to its protracted state – ambiguous loss can last for many years – it can be especially challenging to process difficult feelings because resolution typically occurs only after the person has died. Linked to this is another facet of dementia grief, 'receding of the known self'. This refers to losses relating to the abilities, roles, identity and characteristics of the person living with dementia. For some carers, the loss of the known self is associated with profound pre-death grief akin to post-death bereavement experiences including feelings of anger, guilt, sadness and, for some, acceptance. Care for a partner living with more advanced dementia has been described as quasi-bereavement. There is a paradoxical disconnection between the physical self, which is retained (albeit sometimes altered) and the psychological self, which is eroded by dementia.

Blandin and Pepin (2017) propose a theoretical model of dementia grief suggesting that it cycles through three states – separation, liminality and re-emergence – and that these states occur and re-occur throughout the dementia trajectory. They argue that in order for the carer to manage the ongoing grief process, s/he needs to: acknowledge each significant loss as it happens (separation from the present life and antici-pated future life); learn to tolerate the (often) difficult feelings that it generates (existence between a previous state and an emerging one, i.e. liminality) and adapt to the reality of the changed situation and relationship (re-emergence). Effective re-emergence is associated with positive adapting behaviours such as learning new ways to communicate with the person living with dementia or engaging with formal support for themselves or their relative, e.g. joining a carers support group. Adaptation is a critical step for the carer in moving on with their caring journey and offering stability. This model offers a unique way to explore the process of dementia caring by placing the carer's experiences within the conceptual framework of grief (Dempsey & Baago, 1998). It may help carers to appreciate the role played by grief in their care-giving journey and inform services regarding the timing and nature of interventions, for example to offer support at specific 'points of loss' and help carers to recognise and manage the ongoing grief process. It may additionally help carers to adjust post bereavement.

Carers of Relatives With Severe Functional Mental Health Problems

Work on dementia carers intersects with emerging work on family carers of relatives with severe (functional) mental health problems. Research suggests that many experience 'chronic sorrow': a theoretical concept describing a 'normal grief response' that is associated with ongoing loss (Eakes, 1995). Three types of loss have been identified: loss of the person such as changes to personality; loss of elements of key relationships such as loss of trust between a parent and child with a mental health problem and loss of the anticipated or planned-for future. These are also reflective of Bury's (1991) description of illness as a fundamental rupture in the fabric of everyday life and of the related disruption of people's narratives about their future and the trajectories of their lives (Engman, 2019). As most adults with severe mental health problems develop symptoms relatively young, the limitations imposed by their condition often disrupt the whole of their adult life course and have a significant impact on the lives and well-being of their families too. The lives of parents of a son or daughter with a severe mental health problem are shaped by care responsibilities and choices are often constrained or truncated (Hoseinzadeh et al., 2022). Choices about parental employment opportunities, for example, may be limited by needing to live close to their adult son or daughter.

Triggers for chronic sorrow include: 'never-ending' care responsibilities, managing crises, comparison with social and developmental norms, deterioration of symptoms, hospital admission, being disregarded by healthcare professionals (as carers or close relatives), worries especially about the future and negative role changes, e.g. from functioning undergraduate student to unemployed young man with very limited prospects. Some commentators construct chronic sorrow as a type of trauma that would benefit from a trauma-informed intervention (Phillips et al., 2022).

End-of-Life and Palliative Carers

There is a third group of carers which, due to their distinctive conceptual status, warrant discussion.

The last two decades have seen increasing attention paid to what constitutes good quality care at the end of life (Bailey et al., 2020). Whilst carers and families are a growing feature of this discourse (as noted earlier in the book), their conceptual status remains opaque (Currow, 2015). Generally, in both research and practice, families are viewed through the lens of the terminally ill patient. Their needs are not synonymous with those of the patient, but they are understood through the conduit of the patient's condition, treatment and wishes (Brown & Walter, 2014). One of the key aims of palliative care is to offer a support system to help the family cope during the patient's illness and their own bereavement after death. The fact that palliative care is a health service, whether provided in a hospice or by a team in the community, amplifies the carers' conceptual and actual alignment with the patient. The language and culture of healthcare has colonised the palliative care arena positioning the carer as a 'relative' or 'family member' and as only being uncoupled from the patient once s/he is dead.

The fact that this population of carers are not (usually) caring for a sustained period distinguishes them from other groups of carers. Their care journey often tends to be intense too. How far they are embedded in a caring role and the extent to which they identify as a 'carer' are moot points. They may also be younger, an issue which reflects the historical nature of the hospice movement; its original focus was younger people with cancer. The fact that dementia is now considered a life-limiting condition and that people with later stage dementia qualify for palliative care raises an interesting conceptual question about where being a 'relative of a patient with a life-limiting condition' ends and being a 'carer' begins. That the palliative care language has shifted from 'terminal illness' to 'life-limiting condition' underpins this shift. A much larger, older and more heterogeneous population of patients, and their families, now come under the umbrella of palliative care. Palliative carers will also be caring for longer if conditions such as dementia and chronic obstructive pulmonary disease (COPD) are considered to be life-limiting conditions. There is, perhaps, a conceptual distinction to be made between the terms 'palliative' and 'end of life'. A recent quality standard on end-of-life care (for adults) developed by the National Institute for Health and Care Excellence (NICE, 2021) defines end of life as, 'people who are likely to die within 12 months'. The standard includes support for families and carers.

It is noteworthy that family carers engaged in palliative care do share some conceptual and experiential terrain with the broader carer population(s). For example, research evidence suggests that palliative carers assume they will act as their relatives' advocate representing their needs and interests; they are often worried about who will adopt this role if anything happens to them (Caswell et al., 2019). There is also growing evidence of a range of negative emotional and physical health consequences (as discussed in Chapter 3). Recent studies in the palliative care field suggest that family carers are conceptualised as part of the formal and informal care network and are simultaneously regarded as 'members of the care team' and 'persons in need of support' in their own right (Ateş et al., 2018, p. 17/18). As definitional boundaries become more porous it is likely that more of the care terrain will become shared between 'carers' and 'palliative carers'. In other words, the issues that may distinguish palliative carers from other groups of carers at the moment are likely to become eroded over time as larger numbers of people are included under the umbrella of end-of-life care. The shift to community-based support, and with it a shift away from hospice-based services, is also likely to reduce specialist support for palliative carers.

A second lens that illuminates the experiences of carers in palliative care is that relating to loss, grief and bereavement. There are a number of well-established conceptual models linked to grief – Kubler-Ross's (1969) is perhaps the best known – and they are widely utilised in the development of services to support bereaved carers. Kubler-Ross (1969) described five common stages of grief: denial, anger, bargaining, depression and acceptance. As would be expected these issues overlap with evidence about former carers and the nature of support services developed to meet their needs. It is noteworthy that most support and advice using the language of loss and bereavement is located in the hospice and palliative care sector, charities relating specifically to bereavement such as Cruse Bereavement Support, or is linked to the condition of the relative who died, for example the Parkinson's Society. It is also employed in the dementia carer discourse as discussed above. The COVID pandemic has obliged the NHS, and other agencies, to engage to a much greater degree with the whole issue of relatives and carers being bereaved due to the much larger number of people dying prematurely. It is difficult to know what the longer-term impact of this unprecedented

event will be on the conceptual status of relatives facing
end-of-life issues or, indeed, on the wider carer's agenda.

UNDERSTANDING THE NATURE OF CARE
AND CARING

Understanding about the nature of care and caring has
developed over the last 30 years. It is useful to briefly reflect
on this evolution in order to capture the changes.

In the UK much of the early theorising about caring came
from feminist studies and sociological perspectives that identified the gendered nature of caring, associating the role of
carer with women's unpaid labour within the home (Finch &
Groves, 1983; Larkin et al., 2019). This body of work
critiqued policies and practices which assumed that women
could, and should, provide care to family members with
dependency needs. As noted above, it also articulated a
distinction between 'caring about' and 'caring for'; the former
involves feelings of concern whilst the latter is about the tasks
of tending (Barnes, 2006; Dalley, 1996).

In the 1980s most research conceptualised care as one
person 'doing care' to another (Ray et al., 2009). This
perspective came to be challenged not only because it was seen
as a white middle-class perspective which failed to recognise
class and race dimensions, but also because it tended to
portray disabled people as dependent, passive and without
agency. It also reinforced power differentials between the
carer and cared-for person (Morris, 1991). This perspective
also contrasted negatively with the burgeoning development
of a rights-based agenda for (mainly) younger adults with
disabilities; this agenda aimed to promote the autonomy and
independence of the disabled person (Oliver, 2013). It

intersected, too, with the development of – what subsequently became known as – the social model of disability (Campbell & Oliver, 1996). This model reframes 'the problem' for people with disabilities as located in the wider environment and socio-political context – for example, poverty, lack of access to paid work, limited access to public buildings, stigma and discrimination – rather than the disability itself.

Since the 1990s caring has been recast as about 'being' as well as 'doing'. It has been increasingly characterised as a dimension of relational interdependence challenging both the bifurcation of dependency vs independency and the carer/cared-for dichotomy (Tanner, 2010). Interdependence means two people being mutually dependent on one another. Bowlby et al. consider that 'giving and receiving care is the embodied manifestation of our interdependency' (2010, p. 38). Kittay (2019) argues that nobody is truly autonomous and that independence as a pure state is neither realistic nor desirable; we are all interdependent in one way or another (Ray et al., 2009). An older man may depend on his daughter to give him a lift to hospital appointments whilst he may look after her son (his grandson) after school three days a week. Caring is 'by its very nature a challenge to the notion that individuals are entirely autonomous and self-supporting' (Tronto, 1993, p. 134).

ETHIC OF CARE

The inherent mutuality and attachment that characterises care relationships has been emphasised in the growing body of literature on an ethic of care. Fisher and Tronto (1990) define an ethic of care as having five core elements:

- Attentiveness (noticing the needs of others, caring about);

- Taking responsibility for making sure care needs are met (caring for);

- Competence that is ensuring that a caring practice is undertaken properly (caregiving work is done);

- Responsiveness (care receiving – having empathy and awareness of the vulnerabilities and responses of the person being cared for and making adjustments to care accordingly) and

- Solidarity (caring with – when an ongoing cycle of care to continue to meet the cared-for person's needs is established). This fifth element was added at a later date (Tronto, 2013).

Sevenhuijsen (1998) added a sixth element – trust and Engster (2007) suggests a seventh – respect.

The ethic of care approach is concerned with promoting understanding of care as an integral part of all human relationships, embedded in the life course, and a product of interdependence and reciprocity (Barnes, 2012). Care is central to the social fabric of society. It binds together families and communities and shapes our lives; it is also universal (Daly & Lewis, 2000). These notions are embodied in the principles underpinning caregiving: obligation, altruism, duty, love and loyalty. Tronto (1993) defines care as both an activity and a disposition; the practice of 'good care' is in her view, essentially, a moral orientation.

This approach challenges the dominant care discourse which tends to conceptualise care as a 'burden'. From the perspective of the ethic of care, the notion of burdensomeness is a way of marginalising older and disabled people and also 'disassociating the young, fit and able-bodied from their own vulnerability and future old age' (Lloyd, 2012, p. 135). It also underscores the fact that all humans are vulnerable; at some stage we all need help from other people. Caregiving and care receiving are integral parts of all personal and social relationships. By locating care inside everybody's life the ethic of care fundamentally challenges the traditional understanding of care relationships as a 'dependent' person needing care from another 'independent' person (Bond-Taylor, 2017). We return to this issue in Chapter 6.

POLITICAL ETHIC OF CARE

Williams (2004) extends the analytical lens of, what became known as critical care theory, by proposing a 'political ethic of care'. This incorporates paid and unpaid care and reframes care activities as being embedded in one's personal and work life, and in space and time. This not only challenges the work ethic, which Williams considers has dominated our thinking about care, but also 'normalises responsibilities for (both) giving and ... receiving care' (2001, p. 489). This perspective emphasises a collectivist approach to care, accommodates a number of different contexts and allows for the supporting and valuing of difference (Barnes, 2012). It also reflects a re-engagement with the feminist ethics of equity, justice and autonomy and with the principles of citizenship (Lloyd, 2006, 2010). We explore these issues in more depth in Chapter 6.

Critical Care Theory and COVID: A Note

Fine and Tronto (2020) suggest that the COVID pandemic demands a re-engagement with critical care theory. Critical care theory's 'historic context was one of social change, in which improvements in population health came to be expected and infectious diseases were, it seemed, a thing of the past' (Fine & Tronto, 2020, p. 302). As infectious diseases are now an increasing threat to human health, including but not solely from COVID, it is important to take account of how patterns of care are impacted. Caring, suddenly and 24/7, for a very ill relative requires a very different set of skills and life adjustments to those of a person with a long-term chronic condition such as dementia. Fine and Tronto (2020) argue that how we go forward depends not only on our under-standing of how family care has been transformed by the pandemic but also on analysis of governmental responses. Countries with robust public health infrastructures did better overall and responded more effectively to the needs of patients and their carers, for example New Zealand. It is important that we build on some of the positive social changes that have developed during the pandemic. For example, greater aware-ness of the experience of losing a close relative in a short space of time. Also, explore ways that public health regimes can take better account of carers in order to protect them, and those they support, from the negative consequences of current, and future, pandemics.

THE SITE OF CARE

Work specifically exploring the site of care, or the place that care takes place, adds another dimension.

Carers' experiences are not only shaped by their moral orientation, social context, personal and relationship biogra-phy but also by the 'sites and spaces' where care occurs (Milligan & Wiles 2010). In 'framing the home as the preferred site of long term care, community care policies have framed the home as a therapeutic landscape' (Egdell, 2013, p.

890). The carer is obliged to negotiate a balance between protecting the home as a private space and engaging with the institutionalised infrastructure of formal care: a new hybrid space. Aids such as hoists and commodes may take over a lounge and family members may be obliged to structure their days around the timetables of nurses or paid carers. This can make a house feel more like a hospital ward than a home and friends may not wish to visit as there is nowhere for them to sit. Aids may also make people feel uncomfortable. Due to increasing care demands and limited access to formal support 'stress, burden and tension are exacerbated' and the role of 'home as a relaxed and meaningful place of restoration' is threatened (Cunningham et al., 2022, p. 649). This developing area of work links with earlier points in this chapter about carer identity and how the role of carer intersects with the care environment.

THE LIFE COURSE AND FAMILY CARE

More recent analysis has conceptualised caring through the lens of the life course. Proponents argue that 'in the context of population ageing family care should be added as a life course domain' (Keating et al., 2019, p. 147). Whilst it is widely accepted that care is a product of reciprocity, evolves over time and is a core dimension of a number of personal relationships, what is striking about existing work is the lack of attention paid to the longitudinal nature of care. For many carers caring is embedded in a long-term, even lifelong, relationship. Keating et al. (2019) have outlined a way to address this deficit. They propose two structural building blocks of family care trajectories: 'care episodes' and their sequencing across time and 'bookends' that delineate the beginning and end of care. Together, they suggest, 'these. . .establish the form of family care trajectories' (p. 151). They present three types of hypothetical care trajectory: generational care trajectory; career care trajectory and serial care trajectory.

The authors define the generational care trajectory as 'episodes of care within high obligation close-kin relationships'; it is typified by cumulative processes of change in relationships with siblings, in marriage and in parental care. Whilst work in these, largely separate, care arenas is well established, what has yet to be explored is how they unfold across a life course. How might a daughter's care of her parent affect her subsequent care of her husband? How might siblings care of their parents be influenced by long-standing patterns in their family of origin?

Career care trajectory is a 'single episode of care of long duration in a close kin relationship'. A key example of this type of care is parental care of a child with a lifelong disability (Haley & Perkins, 2004). Career care may span much of the parent's adult life course often engaging them in ever more complex care activities (Perkins, 2010). The lives of siblings are also profoundly affected by the parental caring role; care affects their life course as well as that of their parents. The third care trajectory – serial care trajectory – is defined as 'multiple episodes of care to diverse care receivers with no . . . predictable sequencing'. Care commitments may be to non-kin as well as kin, ties may be looser and care may be more discretionary in nature. Keating et al. (2019) suggest that this type of carer may be akin to a good neighbour or 'community member who watches out for others'. The patterning of care in this trajectory is characterised by greater capacity for choice, less intensive levels of care and/or an intermittent need for care e.g. when a person has a mental health crisis care is needed but when they are feeling well less (or no) care is needed. Serial care relationships may also extend the range and size of the social network the carer already has. For example, they may make links with new neighbours.

The life course approach can also be used to explore the impact of caring on a carer's later life health outcomes and well-being (Milne, 2020). Although researchers may evaluate the impact of caring in the short or even medium term the life course impact is only explored to a very limited degree. There is some appreciation of the long-term impact of caring on a young carers' life chances, although this lens does not incorporate the more nuanced connectivity issues proposed by Keating et al. (2019) in the framework described above. The long-term impact on parents of caring for a disabled child or the effect parental care in mid-life has on later life health is little explored. A life course perspective also encourages engagement with a 'carer as expert' approach in practice which promotes a focus on caring that is not exclusively about 'difficulties' but 'instead may be grounded in knowledge that is derived from "being a carer"' (Ray et al., 2009, p. 123). This appreciation makes for a very different type of conversation and intervention than a discussion led by assumptions of difficulties and burden. Drawing on a carer's expertise built up over many years is much more likely to result in a positive outcome too.

One of the key issues that the life course framework raises relates to how care and caring is researched. Care tends to be explored as an instrumental activity (noted above), as a one-off episode or set of episodes, and as reflective of familial norms. Researchers struggle to capture the relational nature of care, particularly in a way that has any influence on service commissioners, policymakers and practitioners, and longitudinal work that follows carers over a sustained period of time is rare (Milne & Larkin, 2015). In order for the role and influence of the life course to be made visible research needs to find a new way(s) to explore the care trajectories outlined here and their inherently relational profiles (Fast et al., 2021). Given the potential for life course analysis to illuminate patterns and cumulative outcomes, including those relating to inequality, it is imperative that we develop research methodologies able to capture care trajectories and the temporal evolution of care (Moen & DePasquale, 2017).

CARING, EMOTIONS AND EXPECTATIONS

If care is about 'being' and is an embedded dimension of a, usually lifelong, relationship it is by definition an emotional experience and often a complex one. There are two lenses on caring and emotions: emotion work and feelings relating to caring.

Emotion work is related to emotional labour (discussed above and also later in this chapter). It involves protecting the nature and character of the cared-for person and the care relationship. This may take the form of underplaying how much the carer does and refusing input from formal services; comments such as 'we can manage' and 'he's not that bad, y'know' are examples. For spouses chronic illness is a shared experience – a dyadic journey; couplehood is highly significant. Hyden and Nilsson (2015) call this the 'We-ness' dimension and Hernandez et al. (2019) refer to the dyad as 'a team'. One of the key challenges for couples where one partner has dementia is to be able to retain a 'we' in the face of a deteriorating condition. Work in this field highlights the powerful interconnection between the 'doing of care' and the 'relational nature of caring'. A wife protects her and her husband's marital identity by referring to holidays spent together or a shared interest in gardening. Emotion work reflects both the love she feels for her husband and their shared life as a married couple. These points interleave with the earlier discussion on interdependency and the ethic of care.

Feelings related to caring are often characterised by ambivalence. Feelings may be in conflict; concern about a person may sit alongside resentment, anger, pity and/or loss (see discussion on dementia loss and grief). Fink (2002) observes that care exists on a continuum, which can 'range from love and nurture ... through to abuse and neglect' (p. 147). Twigg (2000) reminds us that the emotions that are often integral to care relationships can be used negatively. For example, a carer may withhold affection as a way of exerting control over the cared-for person. Discussions of care are, inherently, underpinned by a tension between our ideals of caring and the messy realities of human need, frailty and sheer hard work.

An emphasis on the value of family care risks eclipsing acknowledgement of the emotional difficulties many carers face such as stress (See Chapter 3). Feder-Kittay and Feder (2002) make the point that carers often sacrifice their lives and health to provide care in contexts where the cared-for person may not be willing to acknowledge the carer's contribution. In some instances, the cared-for person may be resentful or even abusive towards their carer, e.g. they may resist being helped with washing or bathing or may become violent when they are stopped from leaving the house at 3 a.m. in the morning. It is easy to present care, as an abstract construct, in a rose-tinted light; the realities of caring may be much darker and more challenging.

The desirability of family care is a related issue; it is almost always presented as 'good', 'right' and 'beneficial' for the cared-for person. Family care may not be appropriate and expectations of families also differ: an older parent may not wish his/her daughter to give up her job or life to care for them, whereas for another parent it may be expected or even demanded (Brannen, 2006). The Chinese notion of filial piety, for example, constructs care of elderly parents as a son's (primarily) or daughter's duty (Stajduhar, 2011). Family care may also be of poor quality; how well might an abused wife care for her husband later in life, or a neglected child care for her mother? Not all family relationships are positive and some people are simply not cut out to be a carer. What is expected of carers is also relevant; carers do not exist in a vacuum. Recent cuts to welfare services in the UK, and COVID, have significantly amplified demands on carers. Manthorpe and Iliffe (2016) suggest that the 'effects of poorly resourced care become framed as a moral failure on the part of family carers who may be accused of being abusive or neglectful' when they slip up or make a mistake due to exhaustion or despair (p. 22). This point was made earlier in the book.

FAMILY AND FORMAL CARE: EXPLORING (SOME) INTERSECTIONS

Although our book is not exploring formal or paid care in any depth, it is important to acknowledge some of the conceptual and experiential issues that are shared by both paid and family carers.

The nursing profession lays the greatest claim to base itself on an ethos, or ethic, of care and the architects of the ethic of care approach acknowledge that all those involved in care, whether unpaid or paid, share a core set of values. As with family caring, nursing care is seen as complex, comprising four key elements: behavioural, moral, cognitive and emotional (Kyle, 1995). Elsewhere good quality nursing care has been described as combining proficient technical knowledge, e.g. about symptoms, with considerate basic care, e.g.

personal care skills, and good interpersonal care, e.g. the ability to engage with the patient and carer (Swanson, 1993).

Twigg's (2000, 2006) work exploring the rather hidden nature of what she calls 'bodywork' is also relevant. She highlights a tendency by most employers, and in most research, to sanitise the management of bodily fluids often referring to it rather opaquely as 'personal care'. This aspect of care work, she argues, can be very challenging, requiring physical labour as well as emotional labour (Hochschild, 2012). Care workers may feel obliged to hide disgust when dealing with excrement or urine; they may also need to suppress feelings of frustration and concern that a personal care task is being rushed to meet the timetabled demands of their employer.

The belief that the person receiving care somehow 'matters' and deserves respect and dignity is routinely identified as pivotal to good quality care in all settings (Dening & Milne, 2021). Affective attributes are highly valued, particularly by service users (Turner et al., 2020). Research with people living with dementia and their carers identify communication and relationship building skills, the delivery of nuanced crafted support and care that is sensitive to the protection of the user's dignity, identity and selfhood, as particularly important (Lloyd, 2015; Tanner, 2013). Doing a good job is also associated with 'going the extra mile'. This form of voluntarism – or quasi-formal labour – does not just take the form of doing tasks outside of working hours, but it may also involve affective labour. In her work with home care staff in the US, Stacey (2005) observed that 'within the close confines of the home, many homecare workers report developing strong, emotional ties with service users similar to kinship bonds' (p. 850). Home care workers invested heavily in building these relationships often worrying about their clients when they are not there and phoning them up to make sure they are ok.

Although these ties accrued benefits in the form of increased self-esteem and job satisfaction, they are also costly to the workers in terms of time, money and emotion.

Bolton and Wibberley (2014) argue that the increased rationalisation of paid care labour has squeezed out its affective dimension transforming it into a 'tightly defined, task based, time poor commodity' (p. 684). The affective, but necessary, work of relationship-building is transferred from a formal labour activity to the informal labour process under-taken in the care worker's own time (Baines, 2004). The risks of exploitation, i.e. taking advantage of the emotional commitment of home care workers, is an obvious consequence of this model and reflects long-standing systemic under-resourcing of community based and residential care services. The extent to which this practice is ethically or morally defensible or sustainable in the long term is an important question for policymakers and commissioners of care services. It also raises questions about the status and nature of care work and about staff pay and conditions.

As with family carers there is concern that the physical components of paid care are the only dimensions of care that are recognised in public and professional literature whilst the less tangible and more affective aspects of care – those that matter more to the cared-for person – are paid far less attention (Tanner, 2016). It is ironic that at a time when the value of person-centred care is promoted so actively that the delivery of care has become increasingly task-focussed; the affective and relational components of care are singularly absent from processes such as commissioning. Commissioning priorities tend to be related to the delivery of instrumental care such as bathing, rather than relationship-based care such as social engagement. Similarly, workers skills are those relating to the performance of physical care tasks, e.g. lifting and handling, not communication skills or the ability to relate to an older or disabled person. There is some evidence of limited, but nevertheless visible, recent reprioritisation of the affective dimension of homecare work by some commissioning agencies in the UK. These can be seen, in part, ... 'as a corrective response to inquiries into failings in residential and nursing care, where the qualities of compassion, empathy and respect for service users were found to be sorely lacking' (Turner et al., 2020, p. 2221). There is related evidence that in contexts where care staff know the person they are supporting well, they are more likely to deliver personalised nuanced care that enhances the older person's quality of life and well-being (Tanner, 2010).

One of the most prominent issues that straddles the formal/informal care arena relates to gender; the majority of both family carers and frontline care workers are female. Both groups share a low status; their roles are often unrecognised, are under or unpaid and their work is widely viewed as unskilled (Pickard et al., 2016). Most care-related work takes place in the private domain and is hidden from view. These features both reflect and reinforce gendered norms, particularly the link between the low status of paid care work and women's unpaid labour in the home. These arguments underpin the feminist analysis discussed earlier in this chapter. It is noteworthy that during the early months of the COVID pandemic care work was exposed to the public gaze, particularly in care home settings where disproportionate numbers of preventable deaths occurred (Anand et al., 2022). Despite this, unusually high, level of attention and claims about the 'importance' of care work, the situation in the care sector is worse than ever regarding pay and conditions, recruitment and retention. This speaks to the embedded and persistent nature of gender-related inequalities that characterise care as well as care policy's ideological alignment with the principles of the neo-liberal market (see Box below).

Neoliberalism is an ideological approach commonly used to refer to market-oriented reforms in policies. Reforms include reducing state influence in the economy and encouraging the independent sector to provide services, such as social care services, previously provided by the public sector. Privatisation and austerity measures are key elements of neoliberalism.

HOW ARE CARERS CONCEPTUALISED IN POLICY AND BY SERVICES?

How carers are conceptualised is important as it shapes the nature and direction of policy. In turn, as noted in Chapter 4, policy shapes how formal care is organised and funded, the role of services 'for carers' and who gains access to publicly funded care.

In the 1990s Twigg and Atkin (1994) sought to explore the way service agencies and professionals responded to carers. They argued that professionals tend to adopt one of four implicit models: carers as resources; carers as co-workers; carers as co-clients; and superseded carers, i.e. carers who can do everything and do not need help. Carers as 'experts' is a more recent idea and one that resonates both with the neo-liberal notion of the 'care consumer' (alongside the service users) and the principles of citizenship (See Chapter 6). It is noteworthy that most publicly funded support for dependent relatives is replacement care, i.e. services are offered on the basis of substituting for the carer's role not as supplementary or complementary. The assumption underpinning this allocation model is that carers are 'resources', or at best, 'co-workers', an issue that has been amplified by austerity measures in the 2000s and the more recent pandemic.

Whilst the co-worker sits comfortably with the notion of carer as 'expert' – the possessor of in-depth knowledge of the person with the condition – it simultaneously challenges models of co-working or co-producing with the service user. As Twigg (1993, p. 154) observes 'duality of focus... has to be kept central'; this is often a difficult goal for practitioners to achieve. There is also a tension between expecting carers to provide semi-professional care whilst engaging with the norms and obligations of familial attachment. There are two lines of tension to work with: that between the informal and formal and that between the carer and the user. Both are challenging to incorporate into a model of co-working, particularly in times of austerity (Scourfield, 2005). Note that the construction of 'expert' in this context is as expert on the cared-for person, *not* on the experiences of caring (articulated in the section above regarding the life course). This confirms the conceptual status of the carer as a co-worker rather than as 'user' in their own right or co-client, as envisioned in the 2014 Care Act (see Chapter 4).

Linked work reviewing recent health and care policies intended to promote choice and control for service users and carers suggests ongoing conceptual confusion. Carers' exclusion from decisions about the form and content of their relative's care package suggests that they are primarily conceptualised as a 'resource' (Larkin & Milne, 2014). This view is reinforced by evidence that assessments of service user need are expected to take account of the family carer's contribution *before* eligibility for local authority support is calculated. In other words, what the carer does for their relative is effectively included as part of the overall care package with services only being provided for tasks or roles that the carer does not fulfil.

With reference to direct payments (see Chapter 4) the picture is, if anything, worse. Not only is there evidence that carers do not benefit from the cared-for person's direct payment, but that they are expected to take on additional roles; roles that used to be done by care professionals. These include organising and overseeing input from formal services and managing the cared-for person's budget (Humphries, 2011; Mitchell et al., 2013). The stealthily growing role of family carers is also evident in the increasing expectation that they will do more, and more complex, instrumental care tasks. The provision of formal training is emblematic of this shift. Whilst some commentators would argue that it benefits carers to have access to training such as 'safe lifting and handling' or 'managing incontinence', others suggest that this approach explicitly recruits carers into the workforce, situating them squarely on the fault line between paid care worker and unpaid carer (Sadler & McKevitt, 2013). It also raises (further) questions about their conceptual status and what might, reasonably, be the limitations of their role.

A study by Manthorpe et al., in 2003, explored primary care professionals' views of carers of people with dementia. Using Twigg and Atkin's (1994) typology they identified a clear role for carers as co-workers. This was most often articulated in relationship to medication. Carers' roles included: helping with patient compliance, supervising the taking of medications, recognising side effects, acquiring knowledge regarding dosage and administration and looking after medications. Carers also alerted professionals to changes in symptoms or behaviour of the person living with dementia.

A common thread that service-related models share is that carers are regarded as autonomous individuals, whose needs for support are separate from those of their relative. As discussed earlier, for most carers caring occurs within, and is an intrinsic part of, a relationship (Rand et al., 2022).

Assessments and interventions that focus on carers' needs – routinely constructed as 'difficulties' – often neglect the relational context of caring. Respite care, for example, provides carers with a 'break' from caring rather than providing support for the care relationship (Kartupelis, 2020). This resonates with Barnes's (2012) argument that well-being for both members of a couple should be understood through a dyadic lens. Autonomy may be best understood as 'relational autonomy' (Breheny et al., 2020).

The dichotomised model of carer/cared also ignores mutuality in caring or, what may be termed, co-caring (Parsons et al., 2021). It is increasingly the case that both members of an older couple are living with serious conditions and support one another, often fulfilling complementary roles. For example, a frail husband may be able to guide his wife with dementia around the kitchen and with cooking whilst he keeps his wife safe and advises her regarding mealtimes, daily routines and medications. An older mother living with her middle-aged son with learning disabilities may also co-care; the mother may do the cooking and arrange for medical appointments whilst the son will do the shopping and housework.

Evidence suggests that both internal factors (such as psychological resources) and external factors (such as social and practical resources) make mutual care possible; also that critical events such as a fall or periods of (additional) illness may lead to a crisis situation that results in one member of the dyad becoming more dependent on the other. This threatens the balance and sustainability of the co-caring status quo. For a couple's independence and shared well-being to be promoted, external support needs to be focussed on the needs of the dyad, or 'care unit', not those of the individual (Rand et al., 2022). It is important to note that most married couples, especially older couples, want to remain independent as a couple for as long as possible. Many couples report positive experiences of mutual caring, view their lives and needs as intertwined, and take pride in 'managing' the challenges that age-related ill health bring together (Hernandez et al., 2019). Alternative models of health and social care support that incorporate a more dyadic perspective are needed to support co-caring more effectively.

CONCLUDING COMMENTS

In this chapter we have offered an overview of the key conceptual and theoretical influences on care, carers and caring. It can best be characterised as a jigsaw of contributions drawn from a number of different subject areas, perspectives and lenses of analysis. Caring spans task, role and relationship; it is about labour, emotion and moral orientation; it is delivered in the now and embedded in a lifelong relationship; and it is both a private activity and the (limited) focus of public policy concern. Care and caring both defy definition and demand it. We cannot respond to the needs of carers or articulate the complexities of care if we do not describe and map out the contours of the conceptual territory.

A number of inequality issues are embedded in this chapter. Gender is highlighted as a cross-cutting dimension of paid and unpaid care; it is also situated at the core of feminist analysis of care and caring. Family care remains one of the primary ways in which gendered inequalities are reinforced and perpetuated. COVID has amplified this tendency. The multiple caring roles that, often, older spouses undertake encompassing instrumental and affective components are also a facet of inequality. The multi-faceted, nuanced and relational nature of these roles tends to go unnoticed, hidden from public view. The growing demands being placed on carers raises the uncomfortable sceptre of exploitation of carers and how far expectations of the 'family' to provide care can be extended. As the welfare state shrinks yet further and carers step into the ever-widening care gap, questions about social justice, carers as citizens and carers' human rights are raised. We explore these issues in Chapter 6.

6

SOCIAL JUSTICE, SOCIAL CITIZENSHIP AND RIGHTS FOR CARERS

INTRODUCTION

Chapter 5 explored how we think about and understand care and caring. In Chapter 6 we turn our attention towards the development of a fairer more just world for carers; we explicitly address the inequalities that have been discussed in earlier chapters.

In order to do this we draw on three key concepts – social justice, social citizenship and rights – and explore the nature of carers' current relationship with them. We also discuss how they might be deployed to develop a 'care-full' system, i.e. a system that places care at its core. There is a vast literature on these topics and, potentially, a great deal to review that is of relevance. We are obliged, for reasons of brevity and coherence, to focus on those issues that have the greatest resonance with the issues we have discussed in the book and to the contemporary lives of carers. This inevitably means that we are saying more about some concepts and issues than others. It is important to acknowledge that much of the material in this chapter, like that in Chapter 5, is academic in nature. It is also more explicitly political in tone. The inequalities that penetrate the world of care and damage the lives of carers are squarely matters of social justice and rights.

We offer boxed definitions of the three key concepts at the start of the relevant section. Examples of how issues or concepts 'land' in the lives and experiences of carers are offered where helpful.

CARERS AND SOCIAL JUSTICE: EXPLORING CONNECTIONS

Social justice refers to a political and philosophical theory that focuses on the concept of fairness in relations between individuals in society and equal access to wealth, opportunities, health care and social privileges. The five main principles of social justice are: access to resources, equity, participation, diversity and human rights. Justice is the concept of fairness. Social justice is fairness as it manifests in society.

The relationship between care and social justice is complex. How the two concepts intersect has been the focus of substantive debate over many years. Whilst articulating the relationship is challenging, a distinctive set of lenses connecting social justice and care have emerged; these are discussed in the following section.

CARE ETHICISTS

Care ethicists have made the strongest, and best-established case, for care and justice to be recognised not as conceptual alternatives but as complementary bedfellows (Gilligan, 2003;

Robinson, 2015). How this complementarity should be made meaningful takes a number of forms; it is also a developing area of enquiry. Ethics of care proponents are concerned with promoting an understanding of care as an integral part of human relationships and a product of interdependence and reciprocity (as discussed in Chapter 5). They emphatically define both vulnerability and care – by which they mean the ways we respond to vulnerability – as political concerns. Once we accept that vulnerability is part of the human condition, i.e. we are all at risk of becoming vulnerable and in need of care at some stage in our lives, the relationship between justice and care becomes an obvious one of 'compatibility and complementarity' (Tronto, 1993, p. 167). If you break your leg, you need your family to help you to take a bath or shower; in a reciprocal way you will help your relative out if they break their leg. Although the need for care in this example is temporary, as is the state of vulnerability, imagine if you needed help in the long term after a road traffic accident or a stroke.

In *Love's Labour* Kittay (2019) accentuated the complimentarity between justice and care by reformulating a well-established theory of justice and adding 'care' to the basket of what the social justice theorist – Rawls – called 'social primary goods' (1999). Social primary goods are distributed by 'the basic structures of society' and include rights (civil rights and political rights), liberties, and income and wealth. They are distributed unevenly; some groups are advantaged by the distribution, others are disadvantaged. Some people are born into a wealthy family for example, whilst others are born into poverty. Some people live in a democratic society and have rights, others live in an oppressive regime and have few or no rights.

By adding care to this list Kittay (2019) is engaging with the concept of 'distributive justice', i.e that resources are allocated on a fair or just basis. Distributive justice is based on three principles: equality, proportionality and fairness. We return to this concept later in the chapter. She is also engaging with the mechanisms of inequality that underpin the care arena, including structural inequalities such as gender and age, and economic and social inequalities such as poverty, and highly rationed publicly funded services. We know from earlier chapters that: carers are more likely to be female, that many long-term carers live in persistent poverty and have (often linked) poor health outcomes, and that access to publicly funded support for both carers and their relative has been radically reduced in the last 20 years. The need to redistribute care-related resources – services, employment rights, welfare benefits – to reduce health and financial risks falling on women and poorer carers is one of the ways of making visible the connection between care and justice.

Kittay (2019) makes a second related argument. She suggests that social justice can only be achieved when '... care is publicly acknowledged as a "good" which society *as a whole* bears a responsibility to provide in a manner that is just to all' (Kittay, 2019, p. 109). This demands societal recognition that we are *all* responsible for each other's well-being and *for* the care of those who are vulnerable and their families (Sevenhuijsen, 1998). Only through accepting collective responsibility for care and embedding this into the infrastructure of care and support, can a society avoid the risks of privatising and marginalising care, devaluing caring as a role, stigmatising the need for care and reinforcing existing inequalities. In other words, we either accept that giving and receiving care is part of all of our lives and thus our collective responsibility to recognise, fund and support, or we leave it up to families and individuals to provide care on their own relying (mainly) on private human and financial resources. It is worth reminding ourselves that those with the fewest resources tend to be particularly disadvantaged by the privatised model.

Kittay's (2019) calls for a 'renewed notion of social justice' incorporating *both* the concept of care *and* the concept of justice. It is important to have both for a number of reasons. Whilst care is centred on maintaining relationships and responding to needs, justice prioritises weighing up costs and benefits, and the relevance of rights and rules (Calder, 2015; Engster, 2007). To paraphrase Held (2006), the justice motive is about fairness and rights whilst the care motive sees that needs are met. In the context of social policy, '… justice is widely regarded as the moral framework for public life, whilst care is seen as the moral framework for private life' (Lloyd, 2012, p. 6). Although there is emerging acceptance that principles of justice should sometimes apply in the private domain of care, for example around issues of domestic abuse, they are not natural allies (see next section). There is a tendency to assign care and justice to falsely dichotomous ethical starting points; it is precisely this boundary that the ethic of care approach disrupts and reconfigures.

CARE-RELATED ISSUES

There are two important ways in which bringing care and justice together can aid understanding of care and caring. As both care and justice risk being rather abstract concepts illustrating how justice may actually inform care is helpful. Here we offer three case examples that make justice a (more) visible dimension of care. The first two are individual cases whilst the third is a care-related decision.

Abuse and Care

Without a commitment to social justice an ethic of care approach might be seen to support a harmful or abusive relationship whilst applying the concept of justice without reference to care risks paying 'no attention to the weight of care obligation, the uneven distribution of care responsibilities or lack of access to care services' (Herring, 2013, p. 67). In other words, both are needed to ensure care is just and justice is care-full (see later in chapter).

Case Example 1: Tom and Betty

An older husband, Tom, gives his wife, Betty, two extra sleeping pills one night because he is exhausted and is desperate to get an unbroken night's sleep. He has also forgotten whether he has already given her the 'usual dose of one tablet' or not. Betty has advanced dementia. She nearly always wakes up several times in the night, regularly wanders around the house and accuses Tom loudly and aggressively of 'keeping her locked up'. As a result of the extra pills Betty struggles to wake up, is very unsteady on her feet and trips and falls. She is admitted to hospital. The local authority and the police are called by the hospital because there is concern that Tom has tried to give his wife an overdose deliberately. In this example we need to weigh up the issue of justice – did Tom mean to harm Betty – with the issue of care – he has looked after his wife devotedly for over 10 years and loves her very much. Betty also wants to stay at home with her husband of 50 years. The local authority has recently reduced Betty's care package from attending an Alzheimer's Society day centre three times a week, to only once a week as it is struggling to balance its books.

Case Example 2: Geoff and Jean

Geoff is 55 years old and lives with his mother Jean. He has a long-term depressive illness. He has taken advantage of Jean's financial generosity and hospitality for many years. When Jean becomes frail in her mid-80s Geoff is expected to provide support. He gains access to Jean's bank account and spends her money on take-aways, booze and nights out. He threatens that he will 'put Jean into a home' if she complains to anyone about this and has, more than once, locked Jean in her bedroom to stop her going out or using the phone (the landline is downstairs). In this example the issue of justice – Jean has a right not be abused and to feel safe in her own home – and the issue of care – Jean needs high-quality care and support that she chooses – co-exist. It may also be unjust that Geoff is assumed to be able, and willing, to look after his mother.

Choosing a Care Home

There are differences between an 'ethic of care' approach and an 'ethic of justice' approach to decisions relating to the use of services. This is illustrated well by what matters in terms of choosing a care home for an older relative (See Case Example 3). In reality most people adopt a mix of the two approaches, but it is helpful to be aware of the ethical location of key priorities.

Barnes (2012) suggests that foregrounding a social justice framework also offers an opportunity for health and social care professionals to address social and economic inequalities and engage with systemic structures that contribute to poor outcomes for carers. Addressing poverty is key as it is a

Case Example 3: Care Home Admission

The ethic of justice perspective demands that decisions are made from a position of interpersonal detachment and objectivity. Choosing the 'best' care home is based on the care home's ratings by the Care Quality Commission,[1] the range and quality of facilities, costs and mealtime options. In contrast, those who approach this choice from the perspective of an ethic of care will prioritise preserving key relationships, such as that between the older person and their family carer, take account of the feelings and views of the older person, appreciate that this decision is complex and emotive and engage with how well the care home meets the psychological needs of residents as well as their physical needs. Whilst there are elements of both perspectives that are useful in coming to a decision, what is prioritised is different according to whether one aligns with an ethic of care or an ethic of justice approach.

fundamental cause of carer harm; 'having less money means a lack of freedom to choose the terms on which the carer role plays out' (Cheshire-Allen & Calder, 2022, p. 52). Whilst this is clearly a policy issue, there is also a role for practitioners in terms of engaging with carer concerns, including those relating to poverty, advocating for services for the carer and their relative and engaging with an honest empathic discussion about whether the carer wishes to, and can safely,

---

1 The Care Quality Commission was established in 2009 to regulate and inspect health and social care providers in England.

continue to provide care. The fact that we now demand more of carers than ever before and provide less support exacerbates these risks. Without paying attention to structural issues there is a risk that practitioners confirm existing gendered, and other, inequalities and deepen disadvantage. There is also the potential to unwittingly collude with, perhaps even encourage, the exploitation of carers.

A Note: Modern Societies

Greater engagement with issues of social justice also reflects the way that we live today (in the West at least). As has been noted in earlier chapters, changes in the nature of work, more women entering the workplace, smaller family sizes and the growth of the elderly population have rendered traditional approaches to caring inadequate. There are pressures to work longer hours and for more years and the demands of caring are now significant and very time consuming. It is almost impossible to manage to work *and* provide care for a relative. There are also more older people without children and a higher number of fractured families; the assumed 'supply' of family carers can no longer be guaranteed (Yeandle et al., 2017).

Recognising that most carers need support in order to provide adequate care to their relative assigns government and policymakers a central role in supporting family care in all its shapes and sizes. In other words, there are a number of key socio-demographic drivers that strengthen the case for achieving social justice for carers.

A POLITICAL ETHIC OF CARE

As discussed in Chapter 5, a number of commentators – notably Williams (2004) and Engster (2015) – have extended the analytical lens of an ethic of care by proposing a political ethic of care.

Barnes (2006) suggests that operationalising, i.e. making tangible and visible, a political ethic of care requires three constituencies to be taken account of: the carer and cared-for person; the sociopolitical location of their needs and the system of support that responds to those needs. Exploring these opens up the possibility of change too. If the infrastructure of care is broken, as political ethicists argue, then what needs to be fixed and what might improvements to the system look like? This question is addressed later on in this chapter.

This argument dovetails with that made by Sevenhuijsen (1998) who suggests that explicitly engaging with political issues 'opens up discursive space for deliberating what constitutes *injustice...*' (p. 145). Considering the many ways in which the 'need' for care and support is linked to life course risks arising from social, structural and geographical inequalities, a focus on care and injustice is not only timely but also offers an opportunity to engage with care as a life course issue (see Chapter 5). Sevenhuijsen (1998) describes a system capable of taking into account the situatedness of human needs and the relationality of the processes through which needs are met as a form of 'caring justice'.

Whilst recognition of carer's needs is a prominent dimension of the political ethics of care, a number of demands from other marginalised groups also emerged alongside those of carers in the 1980s and 1990s: equal rights for women; social inclusion for older and disabled people; and the rights of adults with support needs to high-quality care. There were, and remain, a number of tensions between these groups (Williams, 2012). Expectations that women will provide family care conflict with the goals of gender equality and promoting support for carers is considered, by some, to be at odds with the hard-won rights of disabled people to live independently. Disabled people, understandably, resist being constructed as 'burdens' on their families. One way of summing up such differences might be to say that the carer's movement campaigns *for carers*, while the disability movement campaigns *against care* as a construct and a way of living.

In the next two sections we explore how the current policy and care system is influenced by the political agenda and what the shape and nature of a care system(s) that faces towards social justice for carers might look like.

CARERS, POLICY AND THE CARE SYSTEM: THE ROLE OF 'THE POLITICAL'

Care and caring were first identified as political issues in the 1970s and 1980s, bringing carers into the line of public sight and 'legitimising them as the focus of policy intervention' (Williams, 2012, p. 105). It heralded the introduction of a number of carer-related policies, e.g. Carers (Recognition and Services) Act, 1995, and moved carers from the wings of welfare to its centre stage. The UK carers movement, which began in the mid-1960s, both reflected and drove demand for policy recognition and greater investment in services and welfare benefits for carers. It also led to the establishment of a range of third sector carer's organisations providing support to carers on a national or local basis offering advocacy, advice, information and services (see Chapter 4).

As discussed in Chapter 4, carer's policy cannot be viewed as separate from other relevant policies especially those relating to employment, welfare benefits, education, and health and social care. In turn, the whole policymaking system is located in a political context: politicians mould the shape, and drive the direction, of social policies. In the late 1980s and 1990s the rise in influence of neoliberalism on welfare policy began to displace the voices arguing from a social justice perspective. Policies of cost effectiveness, fiscal restraint and the increased role of the private sector in care provision meant that user and carer rights became replaced by the narratives of 'consumer choice', 'autonomy' and 'self-directed care'. In parallel there was a policy shift towards the achievement of 'parity for carers', marked by the introduction of the 2014 Care Act. That the Act was introduced during an era of welfare austerity significantly diluted its capacity to deliver on its aims.

In the 2000s the neoliberal principles of reducing state funding and improving efficiency became, firmly established dimensions of the provision of public services. This had, and continues to have, a number of consequences for carers (Tronto, 2017). A shrinking of the welfare state inevitably expects more of carers, many of whom are women. It has led to rationing of services – what some term 'welfare conditionality': carers and users need to meet ever more stringent conditions to gain access to publicly funded care services and welfare benefits (Carey, 2021). Raising the eligibility criteria for accessing social care services via the local authority is one such example (see Chapter 4). It is noteworthy that those particularly affected by the cuts are the most disadvantaged. Fernandez and colleagues' analysis in 2012/2013 concluded that 'although reduced access to (social care) services affects a lot of older people, the poor will be the biggest losers' (2013, p. 8). As has been identified earlier in the book, carers are subject to a double whammy of rationing: cuts to services for themselves *and* the people they support. The erosion of benefits for carers is part of the neoliberal push to reduce welfare costs too.

Welfare conditionality also contributes to a systemic, and increasing, tendency to prioritise users (the cared-for person) to the detriment of carers positioning them as 'competitors' for scarce public resources. There has been, in effect, a bifurcation of carers and users shifting responses to care needs even further away from a focus on the relational, often dyadic, context of caring and the interdependent nature of need. That welfare conditionality is being pursued by policymakers as an active ideological force compounds these challenges.

One of the key difficulties for users and carers is managing the conflict between the erosion of access to publicly funded services on the one hand and the policy driven narrative of 'empowerment', 'choice' and 'autonomy' on the other. Carey (2021) argues that this tension creates cognitive dissonance; this is a form of stress which occurs when two actions or ideas are psychologically inconsistent or even contradictory. An older person with support needs is told they have more choice in literature about the Care Act and that they are a consumer of care services (Department of Health and Social Care, 2022). However, when they are assessed by their local authority, they find they have very little choice and may, in fact, simply be offered information (e.g. leaflets, a website link) about services which they are expected to arrange for themselves. As discussed in Chapter 4, many service users report facing a bewildering array of information and a complex care system that they struggle to penetrate. That the consumer-oriented model itself fits ill with the needs and situations of most of the people who require publicly funded social care is a related issue. By definition they tend to have complex and multiple needs: the majority of older people will be frail and/or living with dementia, their mental capacity may be compromised and their carer may be an older person with health problems themselves (Lloyd, 2010). As Tanner (2001) observes, there is 'a central contradiction between being "in need" and functioning as an autonomous, articulate and solvent consumer' (p. 266).

Direct payments are a specific example of a mechanism that promised much and delivered far less (see Chapter 4). They were heralded by policymakers as a mechanism to free users from the constraints of the local authority, facilitate choice and promote independence. In fact, they often increase user's reliance on their carer. There is also limited evidence that direct payments actually result in improved outcomes (Moran et al., 2012). Further, due to welfare conditionality, fewer and fewer people are eligible for direct payments and they are considerably smaller than they were a decade ago.

As Lloyd (2012) wryly observes, whilst the *language of* policy is often highly ambitious and moral in tone, policies in *practice* become subsumed into the political arena where the management of resources is the primary consideration. Micro-level interpersonal relationships are treated as if they are unconnected to the wider social and economic world and to the power differentials embedded in it. They are presented as quite separate from the macro policy, socio-political and societal context that shapes the nature of care, funding issues and how people who need care and support and family carers are perceived and supported. Some commentators would even argue that increasing reliance on family care is part of the neoliberal agenda in health and social care; in other words, expecting more of carers is an overt dimension of 'efficiency' and 'reducing dependency on publicly funded care' (Milne, 2020). This is a similar point to that made above regarding welfare conditionality. It also reinforces the political right's ideological alignment of 'care' with 'the family', already discussed. As noted in Chapter 5, a third more pernicious issue has also emerged, whereby responsibility for poorly resourced care is transferred onto stressed and tired family carers (See Case Example 1 above, Tom and Betty).

A Note: Benefits of the Market for Carers

It is important to recognise that some dimensions of the market ideology did deliver positive outcomes for carers. The 'social investment approach' – policies designed to strengthen people's skills and support them to participate fully in employment – was used by Carers UK[2] as a mechanism to engage with central and local government, work in partnership with employers and secure employment rights for carers (Starr & Szebehely, 2017). Whilst Carers UK's capacity to engage with a labour activation discourse has met some social justice claims, for example improvements for working carers, an ethic of care is largely subordinated to an ethic of work. The broader goal of achieving social justice for *all carers* has yet to be realised (Williams, 2012, 2018).

The political shift that has taken place over the last 20 years, accelerated and amplified in the last 10, has moved the care infrastructure a long way away from any commitment to social justice. How we might redesign the system to face towards justice, fairness and equality for carers, and those they support, is the focus of the next section.

PROMOTING JUSTICE, FAIRNESS AND RIGHTS FOR CARERS

Consideration of the relationship between care and justice raises the question of how carers can best be supported to enable them to make choices and, if they wish to, continue to provide care without disadvantage. Kittay (2019), Tronto (2017), and Barnes (2011) – and others – argue that in order

---

2 Carers UK is a UK wide organisation that campaigns for carers rights, offers advice and information and supports carers.

for carers to provide high-quality care to their relatives, they need to be cared for and to have their own needs met. The centrality of care to health pertains to the health of both the care recipient and the carer; the need to care, as well as the need for care, is fundamental to individual and societal well-being. Care needs to be regarded as politically and economically central to the sustainability of society if we are to achieve social justice for carers.

In Chapter 5 we outlined Tronto's (1993) model of an 'ethic of care': its five elements are attentiveness, responsibility, competence, responsiveness and solidarity. For these to be meaningfully operationalised, responsibility for delivering them needs to be shared with the welfare state. For example, competence does not mean merely ensuring that individual carers are 'trained to care effectively'; it means the necessary resources being available to ensure that carers are able to carry out their role competently, safely and without risk of harm to themselves or the person they are looking after. Also, responsiveness by the carer depends on them having access to timely and agile services that bend and flex to accommodate the changing needs of the cared-for person and the care context. An ethic of care approach makes public support for care activities an intrinsic dimension of social justice.

Morgan (2018) offers a related but different perspective, suggesting that conceptualising and treating family care as a 'social risk' may provide carers with a level of 'social protection' against, at least some, care-related harms. She explicitly recognises the need to engage with issues of justice and fairness. In broad terms, a social risk can be recognised by the state, e.g. the local authority, and social protections offered, for example care services, welfare payments and rights to remain in paid work, or it can be privatised to be carried by the individual and their family. As already discussed, the neo-liberal political turn has shifted risk from the former 'shared' model to the privatised model with, often significant, negative health-related and financial consequences for families and carers.

To qualify as a social risk an issue, or group of people, must share the following characteristics:

- The well-being of the bearer – in this case a family carer – is undermined by a set of negative circumstances that (may) place them at risk of poverty and/or ill health

- The issue, i.e. care and caring, is a universal one

- The risk (related to caring) is unpredictable at the individual level and

- It is a condition or status that the state has taken *some* 'explicit responsibility' for by undertaking *some* kind of 'substantive policy intervention' (e.g. Care Act 2014: see Chapter 4).

Not only do carers qualify as a social risk because they share these key characteristics but also on process grounds, i.e. that the process of caring damages individuals, communities *and* wider society (Morgan, 2018). There is, for example, growing evidence that caring threatens the prosperity of the UK economy. Many mid-life carers are obliged to leave paid work prematurely, undermining the productivity and profitability of their employer's business and reducing their own incomes and (future) pensions. Often, they are at the pinnacle of their careers when care demands arise and they take a great deal of knowledge and expertise with them when they leave paid work to become a carer. Also, the fact that many carers damage their health as a consequence of caring creates additional demands on the health and care system.

Some of this terrain overlaps with the childcare landscape of the 1960s and 1970s. Arguments about women's compromised earning potential, lost career opportunities and the overall health of the economy underpinned the introduction of subsidised nursery costs and parental leave, i.e. parents have a statutory right to up to 18 weeks unpaid leave for each child they have up to the age of 18 years. These social protections are now widely accepted as beneficial for us all, not just for parents, and as a matter of moral and legal rights. Like childcare, caring involves two people: both members of the dyad can place the other at risk of harm (see Tom and Betty). Unlike the support of children and their parents, however, supporting (adult) carers is not regarded as 'everyone's responsibility' nor is it viewed as an investment in the common good of society or the health of its citizens. Work is emerging which identifies care as a social determinant of health and carers as a population at risk of poor physical and mental health outcomes (Public Health England, 2021).

Conceptualising caring as a social risk would enhance its status, foreground a need to pay care much more attention as a collective societal and state responsibility and bring it squarely into the social justice arena. One of the reasons this does not happen is that most carers are women and caring is (usually) located in the private domain of the household. This argument reinforces the call to engage with the feminist infused ethics of care approach and address gendered related inequalities linked to care and caring (Lloyd, 2010).

THE CARE ARENA: INJUSTICES AND INEQUALITIES

One of the fundamental challenges of engaging with a social justice agenda is recognising, and addressing, the role played by social and structural inequalities in creating and amplifying the health problems and disabilities experienced by the populations who need care and support. This is a particularly marked tendency in relationship to older people, who make up the majority of care recipients (Milne, 2020). Poverty is a prominent example. Older people exposed to socio-economic disadvantage across their life course, including in later life itself, are at significantly higher risk of becoming ill and/or frail at a much earlier chronological age than their better-off counterparts (See Graph 6.1). There is some evidence that this is the case for dementia too (Livingston et al., 2020).

Axiomatically, this 'at risk' population tends to require care at an earlier age too, thus implicating family carers in the inequalities that create and sustain chronic illness. As both users and carers in this context tend to be obliged to rely on publicly funded care services, as a consequence of having a low income and few resources, the care system reproduces and deepens disadvantage in the ways outlined above. It also exposes users and carers to a number of systemic injustices. This is illustrated in Case Example 4, Dave and June. Many disabled people and their carers report occupying a stigmatised

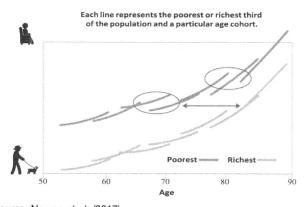

Source: Nazroo et al. (2017).

Graph 6.1. Increase in Frailty for Different Age and Wealth Groups.

status in their communities and in wider society. Being dependent on publicly funded care is also associated with shame and a sense that you have 'failed to provide for yourself'. This sense of failure is deepened by the 'poor lifestyle choices' narrative which has gained considerable traction in recent years, eclipsing that relating to inequalities and life course risks. As Milne (2020) observes, '... the locus of policy rubric (has been) realigned from life course to lifestyle and from structure to individual choice' (p. 133).

Fisher and Tronto (1990) argue that how we think about care is also profoundly affected by inequalities. As we already know from earlier chapters, there is significant variation in

Case Example 4: Dave and June

Dave worked in coal mines all of his adult life. He suffered from 'miners lung' (pneumoconiosis) from his mid-40s and was obliged to retire at 50 years old. He became increasingly disabled and was barely able to walk or bathe himself by his mid-50s. He developed lung cancer too. His wife June – a care worker – was obliged to give up work to care for Dave at age 52 years. They lived on a very low income and relied on welfare benefits to survive. They struggled to access any support from the local authority and as he 'had a family carer' he was not considered a priority. June was reluctant to ask for a carer's assessment believing that she was 'only doing her duty' looking after Dave. Cuts to community services and welfare benefits alongside the cost of living crisis in 2022 meant that they had to start relying on a food bank. They found this shameful; their children were also critical of their parents for relying on 'charity'.

who undertakes caring tasks for how long, how these are distributed and who gains access to support. We have identified gender as a key dimension of inequality in relationship to caring (Lynch et al., 2009). Tronto (2002) suggests that '... the exploitation (of women) is embedded in ... care and family relations' in multiple and complex ways (p. 36). This exploitation takes a number of forms including the expectation that women will: provide care for older and disabled relatives when it is needed, give up paid work to care, care for many years and continue to care in circumstances that damage their own health and well-being. Socio-economically disadvantaged women are at greatest risk. As evidenced in Chapter 3, poverty is both a cause and an effect of caring, especially over the longer term. That women are routinely absent from the arena of political decision-making maintains their invisibility as carers and helps to sustain gender inequality. It also reinforces the division between male decision-makers and the predominantly female profile of those who are impacted by those decisions.

Tronto (2013) views the 'authenticity' of care at the micro level, i.e. the level of the care relationship, as being shaped by macro level, socio-political and economic issues. For example, an elderly wife may struggle to provide the level and quality of care that she knows her husband needs without the support of reliable consistent services. Her wish to do this is compromised by structural issues external to her marriage and home such as very limited access to services. It was this recognition that prompted Tronto (2013) to add 'solidarity' to her original list of elements that make up the ethics of care framework. Adherence to this value not only demands that the injustices and inequalities that undermine the potential for authentic caring are challenged but also that care needs are met in ways 'consistent with (a) commitment to (social) justice' (Brannelly, 2016, p. 307).

A Note: Social Justice, COVID and Carers

The COVID pandemic reminded us all of our human vulnerabilities and our reliance on each other, particularly family members, in a health crisis (Ghandeharian & Fitzgerald, 2022). Research conducted during the first wave of the pandemic captured carers' sense of injustice about their lack of recognition and of their needs being ignored or discounted (Cheshire-Allen & Calder, 2022). Many reported feeling 'dispensable' and 'taken advantage of', simultaneously doing more caring activities and yet feeling even more invisible than before the pandemic. Inadvertently, this was reinforced by the weekly 'clapping for carers' which recognised the role of paid NHS and, to a much lesser degree, social care staff, but *not* family carers. Their role was totally obscured. The pandemic amplified the inequalities associated with caring and how much we, as a society, rely on carers. This reinforces one of our book's central claims, that social justice is a critical issue for carers (Williams, 2018).

CARERS AND (SOCIAL) CITIZENSHIP

Social citizenship is about attaining equality of status, access to economic and social welfare, and having the right to 'live the life of a civilised being according to the standards prevailing in society' (Marshall, 1964, p. 72).

Marshall (1964) – the architect of social citizenship – argued that it requires 'having access to political, civil and social rights'. It goes beyond citizenship, i.e. it is more than having democratic rights as a member of a community or a society. Fundamentally, it is about the relationship between the individual, society and the state. More recent commentators (e.g. Barnes, 2012; Tronto, 2013) argue that by situating matters of care firmly in the public domain, it *becomes* a dimension of citizenship: a care-oriented notion of social citizenship, promoting equality and rights for carers. For example, carers having equal rights with non-carers to an income that protects against poverty, a right to remain in paid work, and to access services that safeguard the carer from becoming ill or exploited due to care demands. Urban and Ward (2020) suggest that one of the prerequisites of good caring is engagement with social citizenship; it is also one of the foundation stones of a political ethic of care (as noted in Chapter 5). These arguments bring social citizenship into alignment with issues of both social justice and of rights (see next section).

Social citizenship also offers, potentially at least, an alternative framework to the neoliberal model of the welfare state. If rights are an intrinsic dimension of social citizenship and social citizenship is an accepted facet of a 'just, pluralistic, democratic society', then carers as citizens should have the opportunity to 'flourish' (Urban & Ward, 2020). Bringing a citizenship lens to bear on carer's lives and contexts does offer a different, much more inclusive, way to (re)conceptualise their relationship to democracy and the state.

Conceptual and applied work in the dementia field may be instructive here. Bartlett and O'Connor (2010) explored the meaning of social citizenship for people living with dementia. They defined it as, 'A relationship, practice or status, in which a person with dementia is entitled to experience freedom from discrimination, and to have opportunities to grow and participate in life to the fullest extent possible' (2010, p. 37). They explicitly recognised that the person with dementia is embedded in, and shaped by, social policies, care practices, socio-structural location (e.g. gender, socio-economic status, race) and conceptualisations of dementia as a condition. These dimensions of experiencing dementia are mirrored in experiences of caring.

Paradoxically, Bartlett and O'Connor's model (2010) struggles to accommodate social citizenship principles for *both* the person living with dementia *and* their carer. Carers occupy an opaque status. However, there are at least two important ways in which the carer's field can learn from this visionary work: that conceptualising social citizenship for a marginalised population with complex needs *is* possible and that caring, much like dementia, is embedded in, and shaped by, a range of socio-structural influences. If it is possible to define social citizenship for people living with dementia, surely it is possible to define it for carers.

CARERS AND (HUMAN) RIGHTS

Rights are legal or ethical principles of freedom or entitlement and *human rights* are the basic rights and freedoms that belong to every person from birth until death. They can be classified as civil, political, economic, social and cultural. There are a number of human rights frameworks including the European Convention on Human Rights.

Globally, caring is increasingly recognised as a human rights issue, particularly for women, and there is a growing call to achieve equality for carers in terms of health outcomes, job opportunities, income and life chances more widely (Hulko et al., 2019).

The extent to which these, largely abstract, goals have been translated into tangible policies or legal provisions is much more muted. On an international basis, there is no United

Nations (UN) Convention on the Rights of Carers. Some commentators argue that existing Conventions, such as the 2008 *Convention on the Rights of Persons with Disabilities (CRPD)*, not only effectively ignore carers but perpetuate a myth of independency that belies a default reliance on them. It '... promotes the individualist fiction rather than the complex, messy, interdependent reality of life' and relationships and, essentially, ignores the fact that many people with complex disabilities depend on their family carer for their survival (Shakespeare et al., 2019, p. 1083).

In a similar way, the 1950 *European Convention on Human Rights* tends to focus on the individual citizen even when where 'the family' is an embedded dimension of a specific human rights Article. Article 8, for example – 'Right to respect for private and family life' – refers to 'the family' as something the individual has a right to have respected; it appears not be worthy of respect per se. That many people struggle to conceptualise the shape and nature of human rights for people with dependency needs is a primary barrier to their operationalisation; this is particularly the case for older people with frailty or dementia. Conceptualising how their carer has human rights is an even greater stretch.

A second barrier relates to ageism. Institutional and structural ageism undermine the definition and delivery of rights for older people including reframing mandatory rights as optional, especially in times of crisis. During the first wave of the pandemic, for example, the human rights of older people living in care homes were flagrantly ignored (Anand et al., 2022). A hugely disproportionate number of older residents died (right to life), many were denied access to their families (Article 8), were exposed to 'inhuman or degrading treatment' (Article 3, e.g. were left to die alone without food, water or comfort) and/or had their 'right to liberty' denied (Article 5, e.g. were locked in their room 24/7).

Residents' families were profoundly affected by these shocking and widespread transgressions. A number successfully sued the government. In April 2022 the UK High Court ruled that 'sending untested patients from hospitals to care homes in early 2020' was unlawful, 'placing vulnerable residents in the path of COVID, leading to premature death and/ or harm'. There is no mention of carers' human, or other, rights in this or related analysis of the care home scandal. For example, their right to visit their relative living in a care home or to have the care home's policy and treatment of the pandemic explained to them. Rights accrue to the individual resident not their carer even if the rights are shared by, or profoundly affect, both parties.

Cahill (2018, 2022) explores the nature of a care and support system for people living with dementia underpinned by human rights principles. Key dimensions include: much more meaningful engagement with people living with dementia in decisions and choices about their care and support; access to appropriate and timely treatments (non-pharmacological as well as pharmacological); access to services including community-based support and long-term care options (such as housing with care models) and involvement of people with dementia and their families in policy development and implementation. There is little mention of carers in any of these; the 'family' is referred to rather opaquely.

The 'off the radar' status of carers in work on rights, including human rights, and social citizenship for people with care and support needs is no accident. It speaks to our ambivalence about where they are situated in relationship to welfare policies; in frameworks to achieve rights for disabled people, older people and people living with dementia; and in the delivery of care. It also speaks to our ignorance about the complexity of care and our discomfort about the significant challenges carers face. These observations resonate with the discussion in Chapter 5 about the tensions that exist around the conceptual status and treatment of carers by services and professionals. Carers tend to be treated as a free resource or a co-worker by agencies not a person with needs for support in their own right. This tendency is amplified by neoliberalism. The market is not amendable to rights; rights are simply not part of its purview.

Thus far, in this chapter, we have explored the relationship between carers and social justice, social citizenship and human rights. A number of key issues emerge. Firstly, it is clear that without a commitment to social justice caring will increasingly be a privatised activity that disadvantages those who do the most and have the least. Care needs to be regarded, and funded, as a public responsibility if carers' health and well-being is to be protected and inequalities addressed. The role of the neoliberal welfare state in (further) reducing access to publicly funded services and welfare benefits for both users and carers highlights the connectivity between political decision-making and social justice. Engaging with the concepts of social citizenship and rights highlights how disadvantaged carers are, how limited their claim on economic, social and human rights is and how little considered they are in the gains that have been achieved for the populations they support.

Analysis reinforces the need for a much bolder shift in thinking, and in action, if we are to genuinely improve the rights, status and well-being of carers. We now turn to discussing what a care-full system could look like if social justice, social citizenship and rights were situated at its core.

DEVELOPING A CARE-FULL SYSTEM

There are a number of elements – building blocks if you will – to designing and developing a care-full system that will deliver for carers (Barnes, 2012). This new system needs to: be underpinned by principles that are drawn from the three concepts we have already explored; be able to offer carers social protection from carer-related risks and inequalities and access to coherent, consistent, collectively funded care and support; prioritise and protect care relationships; and value the work and skills of carers.

KEY PRINCIPLES: RECOGNITION, RIGHTS AND REDISTRIBUTION

Williams (2012, 2018) considers that the following criteria are prerequisites for achieving a socially just system for carers:

- *Recognition*: visibility, voice, respect, dignity

- *Rights*: right to financial and practical support; right to work *and* care; right to social inclusion; right to improved health services and support

- *Redistribution*: of care responsibilities; resources; time

There are four elements to *recognition*. First, is visibility: carers are no longer to be taken for granted, marginalised and/ or ignored. A key point concerns the focus of the 'individual' by the care and support system. Lloyd (2023), quoting Barnes (2006), argues that the 'binary distinction. . .which separates care providers from care-recipients does not reflect the fluid identities and experiences of those involved in caring relationships' (p. 150). Second, is voice: being heard and having the power to influence policies and practices that affect them. Third, is about valuing care: dignity and respect for carers and those they support is essential. *Rights* include rights *as carers* – to work, protect health and well-being and live a life outside caring, *as citizens* (see 'social citizenship' above), and the right to participate. Carers have rights to services too, both for themselves and the person they support.

These principles demand the *redistribution* of care responsibilities, care resources and time. Distributive justice is a key dimension of social justice (Fraser, 2008). At its heart lies fairness: a sharing of the demands of care between the family and the state, in the present and across the life course, and an equitable allocation of care-related resources. This principle intersects with the principle of solidarity noted above.

DIMENSIONS OF A SYSTEM RESTRUCTURE

For these principles to be operationalised, engagement with political and policy decision-making and funding issues is required. If we want improvements in carer's lives, and the lives of their relatives, and to reduce care-related harms and suffering we, as a society, need to accept collective responsibility for care. It demands a shift from the private to the public and from the specific to the wider socio-political context. It also demands a very different policy and system infrastructure than the one we currently have in the UK and in many other developed countries.

Morgan's (2018) aim is to 'ensure (that) all care relationships are provided with comprehensive, consistent and adequate social protection to address their primary care-related risks and eliminate the secondary risks generated by the care... system' itself (p. 193). For this to happen at least two levels of policy intervention are required. Alleviating poverty linked to caring is an obvious risk. This would require funding more, and more generous, welfare benefits for carers and those they support. It would also involve engaging with interventions that would reduce carers falling into poverty, for example, greater incentives for mid-life carers to remain in paid employment. Earlier identification of actual or potential care-related health problems is another way to reduce risk of harm. This may include encouraging primary care services to work in partnership with a 'link worker' from a carer's agency to help identify older spouses who are caring for a partner and parents supporting a son or daughter with a disability and facilitate access to support. Information about caring, for example who carers are, what they do and what support is available, in physical and online spaces, can also help raise awareness.

One of the main problems with the current system is variability. Carers get very different 'offers' from different places and local authority areas. The more deprived an area is, the fewer public services there are. This is called the 'inverse care law'; where there is greatest need, there tends to be the lowest level of support available. An important way to reduce this unevenness is to align local authority eligibility criteria for publicly funded social care. This would provide parity of access to statutory services, i.e. a carer can expect (about) the same level of service wherever they live. The offer also needs to be widened. As noted earlier, carers and their relatives have to have very high levels of 'need' before they are eligible to receive care and support services from their local authority. This not only disadvantages those who rely on their local authority but fails to engage with early intervention opportunities when much more could be achieved by way of prevention, longer term plans made and health risks reduced. A higher level of provision would also alleviate a number of acute risks such as carers and users competing for access to scarce resources and overburdening carers with excessive care demands.

Williams (2012) suggests that well-funded universal ser-vices are also pivotal elements of any care infrastructure. These include accessible leisure facilities, libraries, public transport, and parks. It is not just about good health and social care services: for carers to thrive, have time for them-selves, be able to spend time outside the home alone or with the person they support, meet friends and live a life outside caring, universal services play a key role in promoting health and well-being and reducing risks of poor physical and mental ill health.

A third level of policy intervention is also required: to address the life course related inequalities and risks we out-lined above. Reducing poverty at all life stages is a key example and tackling issues of gender inequality is another. For in-depth analysis of life course risks to late life health – especially mental health – and how to address them, see Milne (2020), particularly the Conclusion.

Of course, many of these suggestions have been thought of by others and attempts have been made to deliver them too (e.g. flexible working for employees who are carers, carers link workers in primary care) but not consistently, over the longer term, or evenly across the country. Sufficient, sustainable public funding is a key requirement of any new care system that delivers improvements for carers and reduces social risk. Engster (2007) concurs arguing that the central role of a 'revised welfare state is. . . to provide public support for caring activities' (p. 13). Williams (2004) goes further suggesting that the state needs to 'guarantee' access to care and support when it is needed whether you are giving or receiving care; she places particular emphasis on ensuring sufficient time for care. The purposeful employment of more rights-based language – in place of care-oriented language – has also been identified as important. It engages with notions of entitlement and justice. There is evidence that older people and their carers find it easier to ask for, and access, services if they perceive themselves to have a legal and legitimate 'right' to them rather than a 'need' for them (Bartlett & O'Connor, 2010). This point links with arguments about human rights made above.

CARE AND RELATIONSHIPS

Across the whole book, particularly Chapter 5, we have highlighted the fact that care is an integral part of all human relationships, embedded in the life course, and a product of interdependence and reciprocity. Relationships are central to care, they lie at its core, and constitute the basis for care. It is for these reasons that relationships need to permeate (the new) care-full system. Much greater time and attention needs to be given to care relationships; they need to be appreciated and nurtured (Williams, 2012).

We also discussed the emotional labour that carers are routinely involved in to support the care dyad and protect the cared-for person's dignity, role and status. Carers are required to manage their own emotional reactions to their changed situation, the deteriorating health of their relative and the demands of caring. This is complex and often challenging terrain. Yet most services construct care as instrumental or practical and although carers agencies may offer support groups and peer support, the emotional and psychological dimensions of caring and the changes to the relationship contingent upon ill health are barely acknowledged. It is these changes that carers first become aware of, not a need for personal care or mobility problems.

If services adopted a relational lens on the care situation from the start, a different set of responses would need to be offered. This might include: family or couples therapy, nuanced psychological support, counselling, cognitive behavioural therapy or trauma-informed care (Henderson & Forbat, 2002). Psychological services for carers, if offered at all, tend to be offered late on in the care trajectory often with a focus on 'coping' or alleviating the symptoms of anxiety or depression. The relationship becomes lost.

We need to reframe the purpose of practice with carers and the person they look after and rethink the role of services. Much more attention needs to be paid to the earlier stages of caring when there are opportunities to offer support to the relationship and promote carer and user well-being. If government claims that it 'recognises the value and importance of the work that carers do', then it needs to invest in services and practices that: prioritise the care relationship; recognise interdependency, mutuality and reciprocity; appreciate the emotional journey that carers are on from the very start of their relative's illness; the need for carers to look after themselves; and understand the lived experiences of the carer and their relative. These are the hallmarks of care-full practice: an approach to practice that reflects the ethic of care framework and aligns with the principle of social justice.

We recognise that all these suggested changes would require a radical revision of the system, policy and services, a commitment to much more public funding and a reversal of the current adherence to the neoliberal model of welfare. Whilst these may be significant, they do not embrace the full implications of a model based on the values and aims of a (political) ethics of care framework. That is for another day. Here we have outlined some of the ways in which the system can be changed and the infrastructure reshaped to face towards risk reduction, improvements to the lives and health of carers, and care practice that recognises the complexity and relational nature of care.

CONCLUDING COMMENTS

In this chapter we have explored the dimensions and nature of
the intersection of carers and caring with the constructs of
social justice, social citizenship and rights, including human
rights. Once we accept that we will all be vulnerable at some
point in our lives and in need of care, caring becomes an issue
we need to pay attention to: shifting care from the private
sphere to the public sphere, from the edges of society to its
centre, from the few to the many, and from something that
concerns only those who give or receive care to everybody. We
have attempted to locate care inside the political domain and
have made visible the need to address the ways in which
caring creates and amplifies inequalities. The case for a
care-full system has also been made placing social justice,
social citizenship and rights at its heart. How we might move
forward and what might the dimensions of a revised more
holistic approach to engaging with care and caring and
reducing risk and inequality is the focus of our final chapter.

7

FINAL REFLECTIONS: LOOKING FORWARD

This book has offered an analysis of the key contours of the family care and caring landscape. It is a huge subject with many tentacles; these reach into practically all aspects of family and community life and intersect with a wide range of social, political and personal issues. Caring is relevant to all families and societies. It is a truly global issue. The authors have drawn together material from the overlapping, but hitherto largely separate, fields of research, policy and services, carer-generated evidence, care theory and work relating to rights and social justice, into a coherent whole. We have attempted to offer the readership an overarching critically informed, yet accessible, understanding of care and caring.

As with any book, there are the inevitable gaps in content. Although the book is primarily focussed on the UK, many of the key threads and arguments will have international relevance. This is particularly the case for more developed countries. Whilst we have not focussed on specific 'types' of carers, we have prioritised inequalities and caring and how particular individuals and groups of carers are disadvantaged by caring. The role played by socio-political issues and the health and care system in amplifying disadvantage has also been foregrounded.

In this last chapter we offer a number of reflections drawing on five overarching issues explored in the book.

CARE, CARING AND CARERS: EXPLORING CONNECTIONS

Firstly, and most fundamentally, care is part of life and permeates the whole of society. We will all need care sooner or later and are very likely to provide it too: many of us will become carers, either in the short or longer term, at some point in our lives (if we are not a carer already). Care and vulnerability are a part of the human condition; they are embedded in our relationships and life course. We care and support our spouses and children and, if we need help in later life, our children often care for us. Once we accept this, perhaps obvious, profile of care, it is a short step to accepting that caring is relevant to everybody. It is not some distant abstract notion that affects other people.

As we have discussed in our book family carers tend to be constructed narrowly; they are a relatively boundaried population of people who look after relatives (usually) who are elderly and frail, disabled or who have chronic physical or mental health problems. This narrative separates out 'us' from 'them' – the 'normals' from the 'carers' – and puts distance between the issues that matter to all of us and the issues that matter to carers. A part of this is about 'disassociating the young, fit and able-bodied from their own vulnerability and future old age' (Lloyd, 2012, p. 135). Whilst we acknowledge that we are *not* all carers – see Chapter 1 for a definition of a carer – care and caring are intrinsic dimensions of our lives and those of our families. There is an inherent contradiction between the idea of care as an activity we are all involved with and the construction of carers in policy.

These connections are important. If care is a universal need and 'to care' is a part of most personal relationships, then it makes sense for responsibility for care provision to be supported as an activity and a role by societal resources. As we have noted, care tends to be viewed as a private, familial responsibility rather than as a 'public good' like health care, a commodity or service that is made available to all members of a society. A second, linked, issue relates to how family care is portrayed in public and policy discourse. The family is not only presented as virtuous, competent and willing but as the 'natural' provider of care for dependent or ill members. A recent example is discussion about ageing without children. Childlessness is framed negatively in terms of increased demands on care services. This narrative reinforces the normative expectation that children 'provide care for their parents'; it also ignores the failure of the state to address care deficits preferring instead to talk about the decreasing 'supply' of family carers (Hall et al., 2022). Policy language about 'the caring family' elides into family members 'becoming carers'. This linguistic sleight of hand tends to go unchallenged. It is bound up with issues of duty and responsibility and with the 'carer as hero' image which, as Lloyd (2023) points out, undermines claims about the need to share care with the welfare state and the rights for carers to be protected from unreasonable care demands.

We have discussed (some of) the consequences of the ever-increasing shift towards expecting more of family carers on their health and well-being. By extension it can be argued that, as a society, we are exploiting carers' willingness to care, knowingly undermining their health and well-being and placing them in situations of physical and/or psychological risk. These risks are amplified in contexts where the carer has few resources and is dependent on the public sector for support. A reframing of risk is the focus of our second issue.

SOCIAL RISK AND SOCIAL PROTECTION

Arguments in favour of treating unpaid care as a social risk were explored in Chapter 5. There are two levels of social risk in the care context: primary risk, i.e. becoming a carer, and secondary risks related to caring such as poverty, exclusion from employment, physical injuries and chronic health problems. Morgan (2018) points out that there are two risk bearers with caring: the cared for person and the carer. The current privatised model leaves both members of the dyad unsupported and expected to make their own care arrangements. Deficiencies in the formal care system, and retrenchment of welfare, have amplified a number of secondary risks and deepened existing inequalities, including those linked to gender, race, age, socio-economic disadvantage and sexuality (Lloyd, 2023; Milne, 2020). This argument dovetails with that made about care as a social determinant of health. As has been made clear in our book, there are a range of non-medical factors that influence who is at risk of becoming a carer and, thereby, who is exposed to the secondary risks related to caring.

Constructing care as an issue requiring social protection would reduce some of these secondary risks. Social protection would be delivered via policies and systems that protect vulnerable individuals and groups – in this case carers – from poverty, harm to health and inequality (Public Health England, 2021). As has been identified, the current system does quite the opposite, it exacerbates the marginalisation and devaluation of unpaid care and amplifies pre-existing inequalities and disadvantage.

In Chapter 6 we suggested that there may be a case for according family care the same social protection status as childcare – namely to regard caring as contributing to societal well-being in the same way as the care of children does – and thereby ensuring access to collectively funded public support and recognition, including a right to an adequate income and paid work. As anyone can become a carer and that caring demands are unpredictable, uncertain, constantly evolving and potentially life-changing qualifies it as an issue that requires social protection. The pooling of risk is also the most socially just model of supporting carers. The COVID pandemic raised new questions about social protection and risk and the relationship between the individual citizen, including carers, and the state; it also reminded us we are all vulnerable and in need of care if we become ill.

In 2010, Carers UK operationalised a model of social protection by developing, what was termed, a 'social contract' for carers. It was, in essence, a contract between society, the health and care infrastructure and carers. Its key dimensions were:

- A nationally determined entitlement to care and support which recognises the contributions of families and carers,

- A funding system for care which is fair and transparent,

- Flexibility and support from employers to provide work-places that meet both business needs and the needs of families and individuals to juggle paid work and care,

- A tax and benefits system which prevents financial hard-ship, recognises families' contribution to care and gives carers the flexibility and security to provide care and remain in paid work and

• Communities which better understand and respond to the impacts of disability, chronic illness, age and caring on people's lives, supported by public services – health, care, transport, housing, education, leisure – that enhance family life (Carers UK, 2010).

Some critics would argue that a social contract for carers needs to be more ambitious than this if it to address the social risks related to caring. Others would say that this contract makes a robust contribution to recognising at least some of the main ways in which carers are exposed to disadvantage and what is needed to address those disadvantages. It is also infused with the principles of rights, entitlements and fairness. What the contract lacked, and still lacks, is the political commitment to deliver on its aims, including funding issues: until these are accepted it will remain, almost entirely, theoretical.

DEMOCRACY AND SOCIAL JUSTICE

Policies on unpaid care have not only fallen woefully short in terms of their capacity to meet the needs of carers but have contributed to carer harm and are responsible, along with under-funding, for the development of an uneven, opaque and inaccessible care and support system (Lloyd, 2023). As discussed in earlier chapters, very high eligibility criteria (for accessing publicly funded care) and the low level of carer and disability related welfare benefits have compounded and deepened pre-existing social and structural inequalities (Senior et al., 2020).

Tronto (2017) argues that the resurgence of families as the 'proper locus of care' is an expected response from neoliberal policy systems; it is the role of the family to care for its elderly and dependent members and to take responsibility for the financial and social implications of care too. The perception, and treatment, of carers as a free background resource is an inevitable consequence of this model; pressure is further amplified in a care crisis where family carers are expected to 'pick up the slack' of the retreating welfare state (Fast et al., 2021; Scourfield, 2005). In this context the primary focus of care and support is overtly on sustaining carers input rather than on the stated policy aims of promoting carers health and well-being, engagement with paid work and the pursuit of 'a life outside caring' (Kirby et al., 2022). This underscores Lloyd's (2012) – previously noted – observation that, whilst the *language of* policies is highly moral in tone, policies in *practice* become subsumed into the political arena where the management of resources is the primary consideration.

As we noted in earlier chapters, the neo-liberal market impacts carers unequally; those with the least are the most disadvantaged. The dependency of services on market forces also puts at risk the long-term security necessary to enable carers to continue to care safely. Carers often rely on one, or more, services with whom they have an established trust relationship; the closure of these services threatens the carer's capacity to continue caring and destabilises their, often fragile, network of support. Despite claims about the role of the market as enhancing the efficiency and flexibility of social care services, evidence suggests that, in many areas, it has profoundly undermined the capacity of services to deliver reliable sustainable support to carers and their relatives (Fine & Tronto, 2020). It is noteworthy that during the COVID pandemic those countries with established public health systems responded much more effectively to the crisis than those whose health-care system was based on market principles, such as the United States (Talic et al., 2021).

A discourse aligned to the principles of social justice and human rights is the most widely accepted alternative to the individualised neo-liberal narrative (Labonté, 2008). A number of key commentators consider that social justice will only be achieved if there is a universal system of support funded out of taxation; a model where responsibility for providing and funding care is shared between families and the welfare state (Pickard, 2012). A sustainable model that can offer social protection – and reduce social risks for both carers and the people they support – can only be delivered via the state as, unlike the market, the state has the capacity to equalise access and ensure provision for all (Stensöta, 2020). Sufficiency of support is also a prerequisite for a fairer and more equitable system. Whilst support may take a number of forms, including more care services for carers and their relatives, higher direct payments and/or increased welfare benefits, a key aim is to ensure carers are not exploited and their health is protected (Thomas, 2007). It is also relevant that one of the main mechanisms governments can deploy to reduce health and social inequalities is to ensure that 'social justice and sustainability are at the heart of all policies' (Marmot et al., 2010, p. 21).

One of the boundaries Tronto (2013) seeks to dismantle is between morality and politics. Her work calls for 'care thinking' to be brought into 'political thinking'. Barnes (2012) agrees arguing for much greater engagement between the informal personal space of giving and receiving care and the formal political space where care policies are deliberated. Care policy is uncoupled from the realities of care. This not only 'obfuscates the way in which political considerations influence and shape' responses (Lloyd, 2012, p. 6) but contributes to the gulf that exists between policy aims and the operationalisation of those aims. A closer connection between the two would, according to Stensöta (2020), help to 'anchor care in democracy' as well as make visible the outcomes of political decision-making (p. 79). It would also help to make visible the ways in which inequalities and care are connected.

THE CARE RELATIONSHIP

It is axiomatically the case that care is part of a relationship; it lies at the very heart of caring. The ethic of care approach is concerned with promoting an understanding of care as an integral part of *all* human relationships, as embedded in the life course, and as a product of interdependence and reciprocity. As noted in earlier chapters care is both about *being* – it reflects feelings such as love, attachment and duty – and is about *doing* – supporting the person with daily activities and care tasks. But care is also about supporting the relationship; carers work hard to retain the relationship's (pre)existing identity and features, reinforce relational roles and bolster rituals and routines. This is a particularly prominent feature of dementia care.

The care system struggles to accommodate the care relationship. 'People with care and support needs' and 'carers' are routinely constructed as separate entities in policy; this is the case in the 2014 Care Act, for example (see Chapter 4). In the 2021 social care white paper – *People at the Heart of Care* – 'personalised care' is presented as best achieved by recognising 'a person as *an individual* with specific needs, wishes and aims' (Department of Health & Social Care, 2021; Marczak et al., 2022). This binary separation does not reflect the fluid identities and experiences of those involved in caring relationships nor its temporality or mutuality. A mother may provide a lot of support to her son with a learning disability when he is a child and young adult: when she is elderly and frail he may provide support to her. Also, spouse carers often provide mutual care and support. The binary narrative also belies the underfunding of care services. Earlier in the book, we discussed the fact that 'carers' and 'users' are, in effect, in competition for scarce public resources, an issue that has been amplified by austerity and welfare conditionality. We are not suggesting carers should not have statutory rights – although they actually have very few – but rather that a balance needs to be struck between gaining rights for one party at the expense of the other. Clough (2014) suggests that care ethics are compatible with a focus on rights so long as the lens of understanding rights, and access to support, accommodates the care relationship not just the individual 'carer' and 'user'. Although we have yet to develop ways to accommodate the care dyad, early evidence suggests that a dyadic approach to assessment of need can yield positive outcomes (Rand et al., 2022). Recalibrating effective support for carers as support for the care dyad significantly challenges existing models of care. It demands a different conceptual frame of reference that reflects the lived experience of carers and a practice that takes account of the nuanced complex reality of providing, and of receiving, care (Rummery & Fine, 2012).

Care relationships have received much less attention in research literature than 'the doing of care' has. There is an emphasis on instrumental care tasks not on work exploring the 'complex relational nature of care' (Dannefer et al., 2008, p. 105). Knowledge about caring tends to be generated from within a particular paradigm: what Milne and Larkin (2015) call the 'gatherers and evaluators' paradigm. This provides evidence of the extent of family caring, who provides care to whom and with what impact; it also focuses on evaluating policy and service efficacy. The alternative paradigm – the 'conceptualisers and theorisers' – explores the conceptual and experiential nature of care including extending understanding about care relationships. It foregrounds an ethic of care approach and the perspectives of carers too. This body of work is less well funded and challenges normative thinking about care, carers and caring including assumptions about the nature of care and care relationships.

Our focus on family caring in this book has, inevitably, required the adoption of a carer purview. At the same time, we have argued for the importance of a relational lens on caring and for a dyadic approach to understanding care needs. A key future challenge for research, policy and practice is to take account of the carer, the cared-for person and the care relationship. As discussed in Chapter 5, the life course approach to research, and theory development, offers a robust and coherent way forward in terms of illuminating: the developmental nature of care relationships over time, the impact of legacies of caring across the life course, temporal links between caring and inequalities, and how the welfare of carers is intertwined with the lives, well-being and resources of the cared for person and others too (Keating et al., 2019).

CARERS' RIGHTS AND EMPOWERMENT

Despite the policy fanfare, especially around the implementation of the 2014 Care Act, carers have few legal rights. The rights that they do have tend to be permissive, i.e. where a public agency like a local authority has a specific duty such as 'meeting a carer's need for support' it is only required to do this if the carer has 'eligible needs' (see Chapter 4). Eligibility is largely determined by criteria which are a mixture of 'level of need' and finances. Although granting (some) rights to carers was a great achievement for campaigning organisations, it has not resolved the problem of inadequate resources for their support or the support of the people being cared for. As rights exist within a political context which determines how those rights are exercised, it is axiomatic that if they are to be meaningful, they need to be funded appropriately (Lloyd, 2023). Carers also need to be brought into the centre of political debate where decisions about the extent and deployment of public resources are made.

History suggests that the existence of a coherent body of research, a theoretical foundation and a powerful political movement are the building blocks of acquiring legislative rights and greater levels of empowerment. Much can be learnt from the disability movement. One of its key drivers was, and still is, its underpinning by a strong theoretical model, namely the social model of disability. This model asserts that it is not impairment itself that causes disability, rather attitudinal, ideological, institutional, structural and material barriers within society. It has not only been instrumental in acting as a lever to achieve rights for disabled people, but it has raised their public profile and provided a platform upon which to make the case for social, political and economic inclusion (House of Lords, 2022).

The fact that the carers movement lacks a shared theoretical foundation restricts its capacity to take forward a political agenda (Barnes, 2006). As this book makes clear – echoing Larkin and Milne's paper of 2014 – there are many theoretical perspectives relating to care and caring, rather than a single dominant perspective. Speaking with a single voice is important too. Whilst 'disabled people' are clearly not a homogeneous group, one of the strengths of the disability movement, historically at least, was that it was driven forward by a specific group: younger adults with physical disabilities. They were also making a clear set of demands regarding: a decent income; rights to access education, leisure and paid employment; representation on relevant boards and bodies; greater choice and control over the nature of support services they receive; greater access to services; co-design of relevant policies and services; and involvement in key decisions about their lives, health and care. It is important to acknowledge that, despite significant gains, many disabled people have *not* achieved these goals and that funding for their care and support has been eroded in recent years. Also, some groups of people with disabilities, e.g. older people, people living with dementia, are marginal to this movement; only latterly have they become engaged in this socio-political arena (Milne, 2020).

The carers movement has a different historical trajectory. In order to strengthen the case for greater recognition and rights, the carers movement has emphasised the shared experiences and challenges of caring. At the same time the needs of particular groups of carers have been championed by carers agencies and by organisations advocating for the cared-for person such as the Alzheimer's Society, Mencap (a UK charity for people with a learning disability), or Age UK. Whilst both strands are critical in 'making the case for carers', a single powerful narrative tends to be stronger and is more likely to be heard. One of the relative weaknesses of the carers movement is its lack of political purchase. As we have discussed in earlier chapters, the extent to which recognition has been achieved is limited; the same is true for rights, they are conjoined issues. There is a case for greater engagement with the 'collective' across the carer diaspora, for more explicitly political demands to be articulated and for the carers movement to grasp the theoretical nettle.

There are a number of, linked, specific barriers too. The language used to describe carers is antithetical to a rights discourse. If carers are to acquire more legally binding comprehensive rights, a challenge to terms such as 'unsung heroes', 'angels' and 'unpaid members of the social care workforce' is required. A heroic narrative makes it possible to place unlimited demands on carers; harm to carers is hidden in the cloak of virtue and in the platitudes of politicians (Kirby et al., 2022). Another issue relates to reluctance amongst many carers to view caring as a political issue. This is a fundamental challenge, particularly when one considers that some people who 'do caring' do not even see themselves as carers (see Chapter 2). That accurate data about 'who provides care' are only captured on a national basis every 10 years via the Census is a deficit too. Whilst we do not have a recipe to achieve carer empowerment, we have offered a number of the key ingredients. Gaining political traction is probably the most important ingredient of all.

CONCLUSION

In this final chapter we have, in essence, attempted to outline the key dimensions of the care debate: understanding and supporting family care as a part of social and community life; appreciating care as embedded in a relationship and a life course; recognising the need to give and receive care as normative; engaging with the conceptual and theoretical location of care; positioning care inside the social justice arena and, importantly, acknowledging that it is an issue that penetrates all of our lives. Care is overtly a political issue as well as a personal and moral one. Caring also intersects with a wide range of social and structural inequalities and has a powerful capacity to amplify pre-existing disadvantage.

The five issues explored in this chapter interleave in myriad ways. This is the nature of care and caring; it defies definition and analysis and yet demands both. We have attempted to bring together evidence from a wide range of different sources and reconcile the conceptual, ideological and political with issues relating to policy and services and the lived experiences of carers. We have also made the case for care to be recognised as a societal issue, and one that warrants public attention and collective universal funding; this positions care and caring squarely inside the political domain. We are in urgent need of a politics that situates care front and centre, not on the periphery (Lloyd, 2023). As care and caring are relevant to all of our relationships, it is critical that we engage with the issues raised in this book. By doing this we advance understanding of care, elevate its importance, 'own care' as part of ordinary life, help to infiltrate the central cortex of political decision-making and make visible the need to protect carers' health and well-being. Caring is everybody's business: we hope our book helps to make it so.

GLOSSARY OF KEY TERMS

Attendance Allowance: Attendance Allowance is a non-contributory welfare benefit that helps fund the extra costs of managing a disability that is severe enough to require support from another person/people.

Austerity: Austerity is a set of political-economic policies that aim to reduce government spending through cuts, tax increases or a combination of both.

Care:

- *Noun:* The provision of what is necessary for the health, welfare, maintenance and protection of someone who needs care
- *Verb:* Feel concern or interest; attach importance to something

Carer: 'Anyone who cares, unpaid, for a friend or family member who due to illness, disability, a mental health problem or an addiction cannot cope without their support' (Carers Trust: https://carers.org/about-caring/aboutcaring).

Carer's Allowance: Carer's Allowance is a non-contributory welfare benefit payable to people who care for a disabled person for at least 35 hours a week.

Carers organisations: These are (usually) third sector agencies that provide support, information and advice to family carers.

Some carers organisations are commissioned by local authorities to conduct assessments of need and other statutory functions.

Caring:

- *Noun:* The work or practice of looking after those who need help to care for themselves, especially on account of age or illness
- *Adjective:* Displaying kindness and concern for others

Commissioning: This term refers to the process whereby a public sector employee (most often from a local authority) commissions (buys) a service from an independent sector provider on behalf of their agency. The provider may be from the private sector or the third sector. Most carers services are provided by the third sector and commissioned by the local authority.

Dyadic relationship: An intimate two-person relationship, often long term in nature.

Eligibility for support: Local authorities have a set of criteria (often broadly constituted) that define the levels and types of care needs that they will fund support for.

Inequality/ies:

Social inequality/ies refer to uneven access to social and economic resources across the life course. These underpin inequalities in health

Structural inequality refers to a system where prevailing social institutions produce, or reinforce, advantages for some groups or individuals and disadvantage others

Means testing: Adults with care and support needs and carers are (often) financially assessed by their local authority; if they have enough money, they will (usually) be expected to contribute to the costs of providing their services.

Paid carer/care worker: Workers who are paid to provide formal care to an older or disabled person who needs help to manage daily living tasks.

Personal budget: A payment given to a service user in lieu of a local authority arranged care package.

Personal care: Help with dressing, bathing, washing, shaving, feeding, using the toilet; physical help with walking, getting up and down stairs, getting into and out of bed; preparing meals, giving, administering and taking medicines and changing dressings.

Personalisation: Personalising services and support to meet the individual needs of adults with care and support needs.

Publicly funded social care: Social care services that are funded – and sometimes provided – by the local authority/local state (in the UK).

Self-funders: People who use their own private resources to pay for care services.

Service user/adults with care and support needs: 'Adults with care and support needs' is the phrase used in the Care Act to describe people who have a right to an assessment of need and/or have their 'eligible needs' met by their local authority.

Social care: The provision of social work, personal care, social support services to children or adults with needs arising from illness, disability or old age, support for carers, protection from abuse or neglect.

REFERENCES

Abbasi-Shavazi, A., Biddle, N., Edwards, B., & Jahromi, M. (2022). Observed effects of the COVID pandemic on the life satisfaction, psychological distress and loneliness of Australian carers and non-carers. *International Journal of Care and Caring*, 6(1), 179–209.

Age UK. (2019). Later life in the United Kingdom 2019. Factsheet. https://www.ageuk.org.uk/our-impact/policy-research/policy-positions/

Al-Janabi, H., Carmichael, F., & Oyebode, J. (2018). Informal care: Choice or constraint? *Scandinavian Journal of Caring Sciences*, 32(1), 157–167.

Aldridge, J. (2008). All work and no play? Understanding the needs of children with caring responsibilities. *Children and Society*, 22(4), 253–264.

Alzheimer's Society. (2020). *From diagnosis to end of life: The lived experiences of dementia care and support*. https://www.alzheimers.org.uk/about-us/policy-and-influencing/from-diagnosis-to-end-of-life

Anand, J., Donnelly, S., Milne, A., Nelson-Becker, H., Vingare, E.-L., Deusdad, B., Cellini, G., Kinni, R.-T., & Pregno, C. (2022). The Covid-19 pandemic & care homes for older people in Europe - Deaths, damage & violations of human rights. *European Journal of Social Work*, 25(5), 804–815.

Argyle, C. (2016). Caring for carers: How community nurses can support carers of people with cancer. *British Journal of Community Nursing, 21*(4), 180–184.

Askey, R., Holmshaw, J., Gamble, C., & Gray, R. (2009). What do carers of people with psychosis need from mental health services? Exploring the views of carers, service users and professionals. *Journal of Family Therapy, 31*(3), 310–331.

Association of Directors of Adult Social Services. (2021). *ADASS activity survey 2021* (pp. 1–18). https://www.adass. org.uk/media/8714/adass-activity-survey-2021-cpdf.pdf

Association of Directors of Adult Social Services. (2022). *Waiting for care and support.* https://www.adass.org.uk/ media/9215/adass-survey-waiting-for-care-support-may-2022-final.pdf

Ateş, G., Ebenau, A. F., Busa, C., Csikos, Á., Hasselaar, J., Jaspers, B., Menten, J., Payne, S., Van Beek, K., Varey, S., Groot, M., & Radbruch, L. (2018). "Never at ease" - Family carers within integrated palliative care: A multinational, mixed method study. *BMC Palliative Care, 17*(39), 1–11.

Austin, A., & Heyes, J. (2020). *Supporting working carers: How employers and employees can benefit.* https://www.cipd. co.uk/Images/supporting-working-carers-2_tcm18-80339.pdf

Bailey, S., Hodgson, D., Lennie, S.-J., Bresnen, M., & Hyde, P. (2020). Managing death: Navigating divergent logics in end of life care. *Sociology of Health & Illness, 42*(6), 1277–1295.

Baines, D. (2004). Caring for nothing: Work organization and unwaged labour in social services. *Work, Employment & Society, 19*(2), 267–295.

Bambra, C., Riordan, R., Ford, J., & Matthews, F. (2020). The COVID pandemic and health inequalities. *Journal of Epidemiology and Community Health*, 74(11), 964–968.

Barnes, M. (2006). *Caring and social justice*. Palgrave Macmillan.

Barnes, M. (2011). Abandoning care? A critical perspective on personalisation from an ethic of care. *Ethics and Social Welfare*, 5(2), 153–167.

Barnes, M. (2012). *Care in everyday life: An ethic of care in practice*. Policy Press.

Bartlett, R., & O'Connor, D. (2010). *Broadening the dementia debate*. Policy Press.

Becker, F., & Becker, S. (2009). Young adult carers in the UK: Experiences, needs and services for carers aged 16–24. *Benefits*, 17(1), 94.

Blair, E., Langdon, K., McIntyre, S., Lawrence, D., & Watson, L. (2019). Survival and mortality in cerebral palsy: Observations to the sixth decade from a data linkage study of a total population register and National Death Index. *BMC Neurology*, 19(1), 1–11.

Blandin, K., & Pepin, R. (2017). Dementia grief: A theoretical model of a unique grief experience. *Dementia*, 16(1), 67–78.

Bolton, S. C., & Wibberley, G. (2014). Domiciliary care: The formal and informal labour process. *Sociology*, 48(4), 682–697.

Bond-Taylor, S. (2017). Tracing an ethic of care in the policy and practice of the troubled families programme. *Social Policy and Society*, 16(1), 131–141.

Bowers, B. J. (1987). Intergenerational caregiving: Adult caregivers and their aging parents. *Advances in Nursing Science*, *9*(2), 20–31.

Bowers, B. J. (1988). Family perceptions of care in a nursing home. *The Gerontologist*, *28*(3), 361–368.

Bowlby, S. R., McKie, L., Gregory, S., & MacPherson, I. (2010). *Interdependency and care over the lifecourse*. Routledge.

Boyle, G. (2020). The moral resilience of young people who care. *Ethics and Social Welfare*, *14*(3), 266–281.

Bradley, E. (2015). Carers and co-production: Enabling expertise through experience? *Mental Health Review Journal*, *20*(4), 232–241.

Brannelly, T. (2016). Citizenship and people living with dementia: A case for the ethics of care. *Dementia*, *15*(3), 304–314.

Brannen, J. (2006). Cultures of intergenerational transmission in four-generation families. *Sociological Review*, *54*(1), 133–154.

Breheny, M., Horrell, B., & Stephens, C. (2020). Caring for older people: Relational narratives of attentiveness, commitment and acceptance. *International Journal of Care and Caring*, *4*(2), 201–214.

Brimblecombe, N., Fernández, J.-L., Knapp, M., Rehill, A., & Wittenberg, R. (2018a). *Unpaid care in England: Future patterns and potential support strategies*. Personal Social Services Research Unit.

Brimblecombe, N., Fernandez, J.-L., Knapp, M., Rehill, A., & Wittenberg, R. (2018b). A review of the international evidence on support for unpaid carers. *Journal of Long Term Care*, 24–40.

Brown, L., & Walter, T. (2014). Towards a social model of end-of-life care. *British Journal of Social Work*, 44(8), 2375–2390.

Buckner, L., & Yeandle, S. (2015). *Valuing carers: The rising value of carers' support*. https://www.carersuk.org/for-professionals/policy/policy-library/valuing-carers-2015

Bunting, M. (2016, March 6). Who will care for us in the future? Watch out for the rise of the robots. *The Guardian*, p. 33.

Burr, V., & Colley, H. (2019). "I just felt as though I had to drop something": The implications of care for female working elder carers' working lives. *Ageing and Society*, 39(5), 877–898.

Bury, M. (1982). Chronic illness as biographical disruption. *Sociology of Health & Illness*, 4(2), 167–182.

Bury, M. (1991). The sociology of chronic illness: A review of research and prospects. *Sociology of Health & Illness*, 13(4), 451–468.

Butt, P. (2020). *Care, poverty, and coronavirus across Britain*. https://policy-practice.oxfam.org/resources/care-poverty-and-coronavirus-across-britain-620980/

Cahill, S. (2018). *Dementia and human rights*. Policy Press.

Cahill, S. (2022). New analytical tools and frameworks to understand dementia: What can a human rights lens offer? *Ageing and Society*, 42(7), 1489–1498.

Calder, G. (2015). Caring about deliberation, deliberating about care. *Ethics and Social Welfare*, 9(2), 130–146.

Campbell, J., & Oliver, M. (1996). *Disability politics: Understanding our past, changing our future*. Routledge.

Carers Trust. (2015). *Supporting students with caring responsibilities*. Carers Trust.

Carers Trust. (2019). *Planning for tomorrow - Supporting older carers who are bereaved or planning for their caring roles to come to an end*. Carers Trust.

Carers Trust. (2022). *Pushed to the edge: Life for unpaid carers in the UK - The voices and experiences of unpaid carers*. Carers Trust.

Carers UK. (2010). *Tipping point for care - Time for a new social contract*. Carers UK.

Carers UK. (2011). *Half a million voices: Improving support for BAME carers*. Carers UK.

Carers UK. (2014). *Carers at breaking point*. https://www.carersuk.org/for-professionals/policy/policy-library/carers-at-breaking-point-report

Carers UK. (2016). *Missing out: The identification challenge*. Carers UK.

Carers UK. (2019a). *Facts about carers 2019. Policy briefing*. Carers UK.

Carers UK. (2019b). *State of caring a snapshot of unpaid care in the UK*. Carers UK.

Carers UK. (2019c). *Juggling work and unpaid care*. Carers UK.

Carers UK. (2020a). *Unseen and undervalued carers: UK pandemic paper*. Carers UK.

Carers UK. (2020b). *Caring behind closed doors*. https://
www.carersuk.org/for-professionals/policy/policy-library/
caring-behind-closed-doors-six-months-on

Carers UK. (2020c). *Carers Week 2020 research report:
Carers during the coronavirus pandemic*. Carers UK.

Carers UK. (2021a). *State of caring 2021: A snapshot of
unpaid care in the UK*. Carers UK.

Carers UK. (2021b). *Breaks or breakdown: Carers Week
report*. Carers UK.

Carers UK. (2022a). *Carers Week 2022 report*. Carers UK.

Carers UK. (2022b). *Under pressure: Caring and the cost of
living crisis*. Carers UK.

Carers UK. (2022c). *Heading for crisis: Caught between
caring and rising costs*. Carers UK.

Carey, M. (2021). Welfare conditionality, ethics and social
care for older people in the UK: From civic rights to
abandonment? *British Journal of Social Work*, *52*(6),
3230–3246.

Cartagena-Farias, J., & Brimblecombe, N. (2022).
Understanding health trajectories among unpaid carers in the
United Kingdom. *Journal of Long Term Care*, 102–113.

Carter, E. (2017). *Supporting young carers in schools: A
toolkit for young carers services*. https://professionals.carers.
org/sites/default/files/supporting_young_carers_in_schools_-_
a_toolkit_for_young_carers_services.pdf

Caswell, G., Hardy, B., Ewing, G., Kennedy, S., & Seymour,
J. (2019). Supporting family carers in home-based end-of-life
care: Using participatory action research to develop a training

programme for support workers and volunteers. *BMJ Supportive & Palliative Care*, 9(1), e4.

Cavaye, J., & Watts, J. H. (2018). Former carers: Issues from the literature. *Families, Relationships and Societies*, 7(1), 141–157.

Centre for Ageing Better. (2021). Living longer: Evidence cards. https://www.ons.gov

Cheesbrough, S., Harding, C., Webster, H., Taylor, L., & Aldridge, J. (2017). *The lives of young carers in England.* Omnibus survey report. Department for Education. https://www.gov.uk/government/uploads/system/uploads/attachment_data/file/582575/Lives_of_young_carers_in_England_Omnibus_research_report.pdf

Cheshire-Allen, M., & Calder, G. (2022). 'No one was clapping for us': Care, social justice and family carer well-being during the COVID pandemic in Wales. *International Journal of Care and Caring*, 6(1), 49–66.

Children's Society. (2020). *The impact of COVID on children and young people.* https://www.childrenssociety.org.uk/information/professionals/resources/impact-of-covid-19-on-young-people

Cipolletta, S., Morandini, B., & Tomaino, S. C. M. (2021). Caring for a person with dementia during the COVID pandemic: A qualitative study with family caregivers. *Ageing and Society*, 1–21.

Clough, B. (2014). What about us? A case for legal recognition of interdependence in informal care relationships. *Journal of Social Welfare and Family Law*, 36(2), 129–148.

Cronin, P., Hynes, G., Breen, M., McCarron, M., McCallion, P., & O'Sullivan, L. (2015). Between worlds: The experiences and needs of former family carers. *Health and Social Care in the Community*, *23*(1), 88–96.

Cunningham, N., Cowie, J., & Methven, K. (2022). Right at home: Living with dementia and multi-morbidities. *Ageing and Society*, *42*(3), 632–656.

Currow, D. (2015). Caregivers' three-cornered hats: Their tricornes. *Palliative Medicine*, *29*(6), 485–486.

Dalley, G. (1996). *Ideologies of caring: Rethinking community and collectivism*. Springer.

Dalton, J., Thomas, S., Harden, M., Eastwood, A., & Parker, G. (2018). Updated meta-review of evidence on support for carers. *Journal of Health Services Research and Policy*, *23*(3), 196–207.

Daly, M., & Lewis, J. (2000). The concept of social care and the analysis of contemporary welfare states. *British Journal of Sociology*, *51*(2), 281–298.

Dannefer, D., Stein, P., Siders, R., & Patterson, R. (2008). Is that all there is? The concept of care and the dialectic of critique. *Journal of Aging Studies*, *22*(2), 101–108.

Davies, S., & Nolan, M. (2004). 'Making the move': Relatives' experiences of the transition to a care home. *Health and Social Care in the Community*, *12*(6), 517–526.

Davies, S., & Nolan, M. (2006). 'Making it better': Self-perceived roles of family caregivers of older people living in care homes: A qualitative study. *International Journal of Nursing Studies*, *43*(3), 281–291.

Dempsey, M., & Baago, S. (1998). Latent grief: The unique and hidden grief of carers of loved ones with dementia. *American Journal of Alzheimer's Disease*, *13*(2), 84–91.

Dening, T., & Milne, A. (2021). Mental health in care homes for older people. In T. Dening, A. Thomas, R. Stewart, & J.-P. Taylor (Eds.), *Oxford textbook of old age psychiatry* (3rd ed., pp. 343–358). Oxford University Press.

Department of Health and Social Care. (2021). *People at the heart of care: Adult social care, reform white paper*. DHSC.

Department of Health and Social Care. (2022). *Care Act: Care and support guidance*. DHSC.

Department for Work and Pensions. (2020). *Family Resources Survey: Financial year 2018/2019*. Office for National Statistics. https://www.gov.uk/government/statistics/family-resources-survey-financial-year-2018-to-2019

Do, E. K., Cohen, S. A., & Brown, M. J. (2014). Socio-economic and demographic factors modify the association between informal caregiving and health in the Sandwich Generation. *BMC Public Health*, *14*(1), 362.

Duncan, K. A., Shooshtari, S., Roger, K., Fast, J., & Han, J. (2020). The cost of caring out-of-pocket expenditures and financial hardship among Canadian carers. *International Journal of Care and Caring*, *4*(2), 141–166.

Eakes, G. (1995). Chronic sorrow: The lived experience of parents of chronically mentally ill individuals. *Archives of Psychiatric Nursing*, *9*(2), 77–84.

Egdell, V. (2013). Who cares? Managing obligation and responsibility across the changing landscapes of informal dementia care. *Ageing and Society*, *33*(5), 888–907.

Embracing Carers. (2021). *The Global Carer Well-Being Index*. https://www.embracingcarers.com/wp-content/uploads/Global-Carer-Well-Being-Index-Report_FINAL.pdf

Engman, A. (2019). Embodiment and the foundation of biographical disruption. *Social Science and Medicine*, *225*, 120–127.

Engster, D. (2007). *The heart of justice: Care ethics and political theory.* Oxford University Press.

Engster, D. (2015). *Justice, care and the welfare state.* Oxford University Press.

Ewing, G., & Grande, G. (2018). *Providing comprehensive, person-centred assessment and support for family carers towards the end of life 10 recommendations for achieving organisational change.* www.hospiceuk.org

Fast, J., Keating, N., Eales, J., Kim, C., & Lee, Y. (2021). Trajectories of family care over the life course: Evidence from Canada. *Ageing and Society*, *41*(5), 1145–1162.

Feder Kittay, E., & Feder, E. K. (Eds.). (2002). *The subject of care: Feminist perspectives on dependency.* Rowman & Littlefield Publishers.

Fernandez, J.-L., Marczak, J., Snell, T., Brimblecombe, N., Moriarty, J., Damant, J., Knapp, M., & Manthorpe, J. (2019). *Supporting carers following the implementation of the Care Act 2014: Eligibility, support and prevention.* Care Policy and Evaluation Centre and Policy Research Unit in Health and Social Care Workforce.

Fernandez, J. L., Snell, T., Forder, J., & Wittenburg, R. (2013). *Implications of setting eligibility criteria for adult social care services in England at the moderate needs level.* Discussion Paper 2851. Personal Social Services Research Unit.

Finch, J., & Groves, D. (Eds.). (1983). *A labour of love: Women, work and caring.* Routledge.

Fine, M., & Tronto, J. (2020). Care goes viral: Care theory and research confront the global covid-19 pandemic. *International Journal of Care and Caring*, 4(3), 301–309.

Fink, J. (2002). Private lives and public issues: Moral panics and 'the family' in 20th century Britain. *Journal for the Study of British Cultures*, 9(2), 135–148.

Fisher, B., & Tronto, J. (1990). Towards a feminist theory of care. In A. Emily & M. Nelson (Eds.), *Circles of care: Work and identity in women's lives* (pp. 36–54). SUNY Press.

Foley, N., Powell, A., Clark, H., Brione, P., Kennedy, S., Powell, T., Roberts, N., Harker, Francis-Devine, B., & Foster, D. (2022). *Informal carers* (pp. 1–64).

Fraser, N. (2008). Reframing justice in a globalizing world. In K. Olson (Ed.), *Adding insult to injury: Nancy Fraser debates her critics* (pp. 273–291). Verso.

Gallagher, S., & Bennett, K. (2021). Caregiving and allostatic load predict future illness and disability: A population-based study. *Brain, Behavior, and Immunity - Health*, 16. https://doi.org/10.1016/j.bbih.2021.100295

Gallagher, S., Daynes-Kearney, R., Bowman-Grangel, A., Dunne, N., & McMahon, J. (2022). Life satisfaction, social participation and symptoms of depression in young adult carers: Evidence from 21 European countries. *International Journal of Adolescence and Youth*, 27(1), 60–71.

Ghandeharian, S., & FitzGerald, M. (2022). COVID-19, the trauma of the 'real' and the political import of vulnerability. *International Journal of Care and Caring*, 6(1/2), 33–47.

Gilligan, C. (2003). *In a different voice: Psychological theory and women's development*. Harvard University Press.

Graham, H. (1991). The concept of caring in feminist research: The case of domestic service. *Sociology*, *25*(1), 61–78.

Greenwood, N., Pound, C., Brearley, S., & Smith, R. (2019). A qualitative study of older informal carers' experiences and perceptions of their caring role. *Maturitas*, *124*, 1–7.

Greenwood, N., & Smith, R. (2019). Motivations for being informal carers of people living with dementia: A systematic review of qualitative literature. *BMC Geriatrics*, *19*(1), 169.

Haley, W. E., & Perkins, E. A. (2004). Current status and future directions in family caregiving and aging people with intellectual disabilities. *Journal of Policy and Practice in Intellectual Disabilities*, *1*(1), 24–30.

Hall, A., Spiers, G., & Hanratty, B. (2022). Constructions of childlessness and ageing: Legitimising dependency on unpaid care? *Quality in Ageing and Older Adults*, *23*(4), 165–173.

Heath, A., Carey, L. B., & Chong, S. (2018). Helping carers care: An Exploratory study of factors impacting informal family carers and their use of aged care services. *Journal of Religion and Health*, *57*(3), 1146–1167.

Held, V. (2006). *The ethics of care: Personal, political, and global*. Oxford University Press.

Henderson, J. (2001). 'He's not my carer - he's my husband': Personal and policy constructions of care in mental health. *Journal of Social Work Practice*, *15*(2), 149–159.

Henderson, J., & Forbat, L. (2002). Relationship-based social policy: Personal and policy constructions of 'care'. *Critical Social Policy*, *22*(4), 669–687.

Hernandez, E., Spencer, B., Ingersoll-Dayton, B., Faber, A., & Ewert, A. (2019). "We are a team": Couple identity and memory loss. *Dementia*, *18*(3), 1166–1180.

Herring, J. (2013). *Caring and the law*. Hart Publishing Ltd.

Hochschild, A. (2012). *The managed heart: Commercialization of human feeling*. University of California Press.

Hoff, A. (2015). *Current and future challenges of family care in the UK: Evidence review*. Future of Ageing. https://www.gov.uk/government/publications/future-of-ageing-volunteering-informal-care-and-paid-work-in-later-life

Hoseinzadeh, F., Miri, S., Foroughameri, G., Farokhzadian, J., & Eslami Shahrbabaki, M. (2022). Stigma, burden of care, and family functioning in family caregivers of people with mental illnesses: A cross-sectional questionnaire survey. *Social Work in Mental Health*, *20*(4), 432–447.

Hounsell, D. (2013). *Hidden from view: The experiences of young carers in England*. The Children's Society.

House of Lords. (2022). *A 'gloriously ordinary life': Spotlight on adult social care*. https://ukparliament.shorthandstories.com/new-deal-adult-social-care-committee-report/index.html

Hughes, B., McKie, L., Hopkins, D., & Watson, N. (2005). Love's labours lost? Feminism, the disabled people's movement and an ethic of care. *Sociology*, *39*(2), 259–275.

Hulko, W., Brotman, S., Stern, L., & Ferrer, I. (2019). *Gerontological work in action: Anti-oppressive practice with older adults, their families, and communities*. Routledge.

Humphries, R. (2011). *Integrating health and social care: Where next?* Kings Fund. https://www.kingsfund.org.uk/publications/integrating-health-and-social-care

Hyden, L. C., & Nilsson, E. (2015). Couples with dementia: Positioning the 'we'. *Dementia*, *14*(6), 716–733.

International Alliance of Carer Organizations. (2021). *Global state of caring*. https://internationalcarers.org/carer-facts/global-carer-stats/

Ipsos Mori. (2021). *GP Patient Survey 2021*. https://www.ipsos.com/en-uk/2021-gp-patient-survey-results-released

Isham, L., Bradbury-Jones, C., & Hewison, A. (2020). Female family carers' experiences of violent, abusive or harmful behaviour by the older person for whom they care: A case of epistemic injustice? *Sociology of Health & Illness*, *42*(1), 80–94.

Jacklin, A. (2021). *Young carers affected by HIV learning report*. The Children's Society.

James, N. (1992). Care = organisation + physical labour + emotional labour. *Sociology of Health & Illness*, *14*(4), 488–509.

James, E. (2019). *Caring alone: Why Black, Asian and Minority Ethnic young carers continue to struggle to access support*. https://www.barnardos.org.uk/sites/default/files/uploads/caring-alone_0.pdf

Kartupelis, J. (2020). *Making relational care work for older people, exploring innovation and best practice in everyday life*. Routledge.

Keady, J., & Nolan, M. (1994). Younger onset dementia: Developing a longitudinal model as the basis for a research agenda and as a guide to interventions with sufferers and carers. *Journal of Advanced Nursing*, *19*(4), 659–669.

Keady, J., & Nolan, M. (2003). The dynamics of dementia: Working together, working separately, or working alone? In

M. Nolan, U. Lundh, G. Grant, & J. Keady (Eds.), *Partnerships in family care: Understanding the caregiving career* (pp. 15–32). Open University Press.

Keating, N., Eales, J., Funk, L., Fast, J., & Min, J. (2019). Life course trajectories of family care. *International Journal of Care and Caring*, 3(2), 147–163.

Keating, N., McGregor, J. A., & Yeandle, S. (2021). Sustainable care: Theorising the well-being of caregivers to older persons. *International Journal of Care and Caring*, 5(4), 611–630.

Kettell, L. (2020). Young adult carers in higher education: The motivations, barriers and challenges involved: A UK study. *Journal of Further and Higher Education*, 44(1), 100–112.

Kings Fund. (2022). *The Health and Care Act: Six key questions*. https://www.kingsfund.org.uk/publications/health-and-care-act-key-questions

Kirby, E., Newton, G., Hofstätter, L., Judd-Lam, S., Strnadová, I., & Newman, C. E. (2022). (How) will it end? A qualitative analysis of free-text survey data on informal care endings. *International Journal of Care and Caring*, 6(4), 604–620.

Kittay, E. (2019). *Love's labor: Essays on women, equality and dependency*. Routledge.

Knowles, S., Combs, R., Kirk, S., Griffiths, M., Patel, N., & Sanders, C. (2016). Hidden caring, hidden carers? Exploring the experience of carers for people with long-term conditions. *Health and Social Care in the Community*, 24(2), 203–213.

Koffman, J., Gross, J., Etkind, S. N., & Selman, L. (2020). Uncertainty and COVID: How are we to respond? *Journal of the Royal Society of Medicine*, 113(6), 211–216.

Kubler-Ross, E. (1969). *On death and dying*. Collier Books/ Macmillan Publishing Co.

Kyle, T. V. (1995). The concept of caring: A review of the literature. *Journal of Advanced Nursing*, *21*(3), 506–514.

Labonté, R. (2008). Global health in public policy: Finding the right frame? *Critical Public Health*, *18*(4), 467–482.

Lafferty, A., Phillips, D., Dowling-Hetherington, L., Fahy, M., Moloney, B., Duffy, C., Paul, G., Fealy, G., & Kroll, T. (2022). Colliding worlds: Family carers' experiences of balancing work and care in Ireland during the COVID pandemic. *Health and Social Care in the Community*, *30*(3), 1133–1142.

Larkin, M. (2009). Life after caring: The post-caring experiences of former carers. *The British Journal of Social Work*, *39*(6), 1026–1042.

Larkin, M. (2011). *Social aspects of health, illness and healthcare*. McGraw-Hill Education.

Larkin, M., Henwood, M., & Milne, A. (2019). Carer-related research and knowledge: Findings from a scoping review. *Health and Social Care in the Community*, *27*(1), 55–67.

Larkin, M., Henwood, M., & Milne, A. (2020). Older carers and carers of people with dementia: Improving and developing effective support. *Social Policy and Society*, *21*(2), 242–256.

Larkin, M., & Kubiak, C. (2021). Carers in higher education: Where next? *Widening Participation and Lifelong Learning*, *23*(2), 130–151.

Larkin, M., & Milne, A. (2014). Carers and empowerment in the UK: A critical reflection. *Social Policy and Society*, *13*(1), 25–38.

Larkin, M., & Milne, A. (2017). What do we know about older former carers? Key issues and themes. *Health and Social Care in the Community*, 25(4), 1396–1403.

Larkin, M., & Milne, A. (2021). Knowledge generation and former carers: Reflections and ways forward. *Families, Relationships and Societies*, 10(2), 287–302.

Larkin, M., & Mitchell, W. (2016). Carers, choice and personalisation: What do we know? *Social Policy and Society*, 15(2), 189–205.

Lewis, F. M., Becker, S., Parkhouse, T., Joseph, S., Hlebec, V., Mrzel, M., Brolin, R., Casu, G., Boccaletti, L., Santini, S., D'Amen, B., Socci, M., Hoefman, R., De Jong, N., Leu, A., Phelps, D., Guggiari, E., Magnusson, L., & Hanson, E. (2023). The first cross-national study of adolescent young carers aged 15–17 in six European countries. *International Journal of Care and Caring*, 7(1), 6–32.

Lewis, J., & Meredith, B. (1989). Contested territory in informal care. In M. Jefferys (Ed.), *Growing old in the twentieth century* (pp. 272–287). Routledge.

Lilleheie, I., Debesay, J., Bye, A., & Bergland, A. (2020). Informal caregivers' views on the quality of healthcare services provided to older patients aged 80 or more in the hospital and 30 days after discharge. *BMC Geriatrics*, 20(1), 1–13.

Livingston, G., Huntley, J., Sommerlad, A., Ames, D., Ballard, C., Banerjee, S., Brayne, C., Burns, A., Cohen-Mansfield, J., Cooper, C., Costafreda, S. G., Dias, A., Fox, N., Gitlin, L. N., Howard, R., Kales, H. C., Kivimäki, M., Larson, E. B., & Ogunniyi, N. (2020). Dementia Prevention, Intervention, and Care: 2020 Report of The Lancet Commission. *Lancet*, 396, 413–446.

Lloyd, L. (2006). A caring profession? The ethics of care and social work with older people. *The British Journal of Social Work*, *36*(7), 1171–1185.

Lloyd, L. (2010). The individual in social care: The ethics of care and the 'personalisation agenda' in services for older people in England. *Ethics and Social Welfare*, *4*(2), 188–200.

Lloyd, L. (2012). *Health and care in ageing societies: A new international approach*. Policy Press.

Lloyd, L. (2015). The fourth age. In J. Twigg & W. Martin (Eds.), *Routledge handbook of cultural gerontology* (pp. 261–268). Routledge.

Lloyd, L. (2023). *Unpaid care policies in the UK: Reflections on rights, resources and relationships*. Policy Press.

Lloyd, J., Patterson, T., & Muers, J. (2016). The positive aspects of caregiving in dementia: A critical review of the qualitative literature. *Dementia*, *15*(6), 1534–1561.

Local Government Association. (2022). *Get in on the Act: Health and Care Act 2022*. https://www.local.gov.uk/publications/get-act-health-and-care-act-2022

Luppi, M., & Nazio, T. (2019). Does gender top family ties? Within-couple and between- sibling sharing of elderly care. *European Sociological Review*, *35*(6), 772–789.

Lynch, K., Baker, J., & Lyons, M. (2009). *Affective equality: Love, care and injustice*. Palgrave Macmillan.

Mahon, A., Tilley, E., Randhawa, G., Pappas, Y., & Vseteckova, J. (2019). Ageing carers and intellectual disability: A scoping review. *Quality in Ageing and Older Adults*, *20*(4), 162–178.

Malli, M. A., Sams, L., Forrester-Jones, R., Murphy, G., & Henwood, M. (2018). Austerity and the lives of people with learning disabilities. A thematic synthesis of current literature. *Disability and Society*, *33*(9), 1412–1435.

Manthorpe, J., & Iliffe, S. (2016). *The dialectics of dementia*. Social Care Workforce Research Unit.

Manthorpe, J., Iliffe, S., & Eden, A. (2003). Testing Twigg and Atkin's typology of caring: A study of primary care professionals' perceptions of dementia care using a modified focus group method. *Health and Social Care in the Community*, *11*(6), 477–485.

Marczak, J., Fernandez, J. L., Manthorpe, J., Brimblecombe, N., Moriarty, J., Knapp, M., & Snell, T. (2022). How have the Care Act 2014 ambitions to support carers translated into local practice? Findings from a process evaluation study of local stakeholders' perceptions of Care Act implementation. *Health & Social Care in the Community*, *30*(5), e1711–e1720.

Marmot, M., Allen, J., Goldblatt, P., Boyce, T., McNeish, D., Grady, M., & Geddes, I. (2010). *Fair society, healthy lives: Strategic review of health inequalities in England post-2010*. The Marmot Review.

Marmot, M., Allen, J., Goldblatt, P., Herd, E., & Morrison, J. (2020). *Build Back Fairer: The COVID-19 Marmot Review. The pandemic, socioeconomic and health inequalities in England*. Institute of Health Equity.

Marshall, T. H. (Ed.). (1964). *Citizenship and social class*. Cambridge University Press.

Mason, J., & Finch, J. (1993). *Negotiating family responsibilities*. Routledge.

Maun, E., Glaser, K., & Corna, L. (2020). Co-resident care-giving and problematic sleep among older people: Evidence from the UK Household Longitudinal Study. *Ageing and Society*, *40*(6), 1195–1222.

McGarry, J. (2009). Defining roles, relationships, boundaries and participation between elderly people and nurses within the home: An ethnographic study. *Health and Social Care in the Community*, *17*(1), 83–91.

Milligan, C., & Wiles, J. (2010). Landscapes of care. *Progress in Human Geography*, *34*(6), 736–754.

Milne, A. (2020). *Mental health in later life, taking a lifecourse approach*. Policy Press.

Milne, A., & Larkin, M. (2015). Knowledge generation about care-giving in the UK: A critical review of research paradigms. *Health and Social Care in the Community*, *23*(1), 4–13.

Mitchell, W., Brooks, J., & Glendinning, C. (2013). *Carers and personalisation: What role do carers play in personalised adult social care? What roles do carers and service users want carers to play?* NIHR School for Social Care Research.

Moen, P., & Depasquale, N. (2017). Family care work: A policy-relevant research agenda. *International Journal of Care and Caring*, *1*(1), 45–62.

Molyneaux, V., Butchard, S., Simpson, J., & Murray, C. (2011). Reconsidering the term 'carer': A critique of the universal adoption of the term 'carer'. *Ageing and Society*, *31*(3), 422–437.

Montgomery, R. J. V., & Kosloski, K. D. (2013). Pathways to a caregiver identity and implications for support services. In R. C. Talley & R. J. V. Montgomery (Eds.), *Caregiving across the lifespan: Research, practice, policy* (pp. 131–156). Springer.

Moore, H., & Gillespie, A. (2014). The caregiving bind: Concealing the demands of informal care can undermine the caregiving identity. *Social Science and Medicine, 116,* 102–109.

Moran, N., Arksey, H., Glendinning, C., Jones, K., Netten, A., & Rabiee, P. (2012). Personalisation and carers: Whose rights? Whose benefits? *The British Journal of Social Work, 42*(3), 461–479.

Morgan, F. (2018). The treatment of informal care-related risks as social risks: An analysis of the English care policy system. *Journal of Social Policy, 47*(1), 179–196.

Morris, J. (1991). "Us" and "them"? Feminist research, community care & disability. *Critical Social Policy, 11*(33), 22–39.

Morris, S. M., King, C., Turner, M., & Payne, S. (2015). Family carers providing support to a person dying in the home setting: A narrative literature review. *Palliative Medicine, 29*(6), 487–495.

Nair, P., Barrado-Martin, Y., Anantqpong, K., Moore, K., Smith, C., Sampson, E., Manthorpe, J., Walters, K., & Davies, N. (2022). Experiences of BAME carers. *Nutrients, 14,* 2395.

National Institute for Health and Care Excellence. (2020). *Supporting adult carers: NICE guideline.* https://www.nice.org.uk/guidance/ng150

National Institute for Health and Care Excellence. (2021). *End of life care for adults, quality standard.* https://www.nice.org.uk/guidance/qs13

Nazroo, J., Bromley, R., & Pendrill, J. (2017). *The golden generation? Wellbeing and inequalities in later life*. Manchester Institute for Collaborative Research on Ageing. http://hummedia.manchester.ac.uk/institutes/micra/news/2017/golden-generation-report-2017.pdf

NHS Digital. (2019). *Personal Social Services Survey of Adult Carers in England*. https://digital.nhs.uk/data-and-information/publications/statistical/personal-social-services-survey-of-adult-carers

NHS England. (2014). *NHS England's commitment to carers*. https://www.england.nhs.uk/wp-content/uploads/2014/05/commitment-to-carers-may14.pdf

Ní Léime, A., Street, D., Vickerstaff, S., Krekula, C., & Loretto, W. (Eds.). (2019). *Gender, ageing and extended working life: Cross national perspectives*. Policy Press.

Nolan, M., Davies, S., & Grant, G. (Eds.). (2001). *Working with older people and their families*. Open University Press.

Nolan, M., Grant, G., & Keady, J. (1996). *Understanding family care: A multidimensional model of caring and coping*. Open University Press.

Nolan, M., Lundh, U., Grant, G., & Keady, J. (Eds.). (2003). *Partnerships in family care: Understanding the caregiving career*. Open University Press.

O'Dwyer, S. T., Janssens, A., Sansom, A., Biddle, L., Mars, B., Slater, T., Moran, P., Stallard, P., Melluish, J., Reakes, L., Walker, A., Andrewartha, C., & Hastings, R. P. (2021). Suicidality in family caregivers of people with long term illnesses and disabilities: A scoping review. *Comprehensive Psychiatry*, *110*. http://doi.org/10.1016/j.comppsych.2021.152261

Office for National Statistics. (2019). *Living longer: Caring in later working life.* https://www.ons.gov.uk/ peoplepopulationandcommunity/birthsdeathsandmarriages/ ageing/artcles/livinglongerhowourpopulationischanging andwhyitmatters/2019-03-15

Office for National Statistics. (2020). *Health and unpaid care question development for Census 2021.* https://www.ons.gov. uk/census/

Office for National Statistics. (2021). *Coronavirus & the social impacts on unpaid carers.* https://www.ons.gov.uk/ peoplepopulationandcommunity/healthandsocialcare/social care/articles/coronavirusandthesocialimpactsonunpaidcare rsingreatbritain/april2021

Office for National Statistics. (2023). Unpaid care, England & Wales, Census 2021. https://www.ons.gov.uk/ peoplepopulationandcommunity/healthandsocialcare/ healthandwellbeing/bulletins/unpaidcareenglandandwales/ census2021

Oldridge, L., & Larkin, M. (2020). Unpaid care: Global growth and policies for sustainability. In W. L. Filho, A. M. Azul, L. Brandli, A. L. Salvia, & T. Wall (Eds.), *Gender equality. Encyclopedia of the UN sustainable development goals.* Springer US.

Oliveira, D., Vass, C., & Aubeeluck, A. (2019). Quality of life on the views of older family carers of people with dementia. *Dementia, 18*(3), 990–1009.

Oliver, M. (2013). The social model of disability: Thirty years on. *Disability and Society, 28*(7), 1024–1026.

O'Neill, A., Gallagher, S., Hannigan, A., & Robinson, K. (2022). Association between work status and depression in informal caregivers: A collaborative modelling approach. *The European Journal of Public Health*, *32*(1), 59–65.

Organisation for Economic Co-operation and Development (2021) *Health at a glance 2021: OECD indicators, informal carers.* https://www.oecd-ilibrary.org/social-issues-migration-health/health-at-a-glance-2021

Overgaard, C., & Mackaway, J. (2022). Kindness as a practice of Kittay's 'doulia' in higher education: Caring for student carers during COVID and beyond. *International Journal of Care and Caring*, *1*(6), 229–245.

Parsons, J. E., Dale, J., MacArtney, J. I., & Nanton, V. (2021). Caring for each other: A rapid review of how mutual dependency is challenged by advanced illness. *International Journal of Care and Caring*, *5*(3), 509–527.

Perkins, E. A. (2010). The compound caregiver: A case study of multiple caregiving roles. *Clinical Gerontologist*, *33*(3), 248–254.

Petrie, K., & Kirkup, J. (2018). *Caring for carers: The lives of family carers in the UK*. The Social Market Foundation.

Phillips, J. (2007). *Care*. Polity.

Phillips, R., Durkin, M., Engward, H., Cable, G., & Iancu, M. (2022). The impact of caring for family members with mental illnesses on the caregiver: A scoping review. *Health Promotion International*, *20*, 1–21

Pickard, S. (2010). The 'good carer': Moral practices in late modernity. *Sociology*, *44*(3), 471–487.

Pickard, L. (2012). Substitution between formal and informal care: A 'natural experiment' in social policy in Britain between 1985 and 2000. *Ageing and Society*, *32*(7), 1147–1175.

Pickard, S., & Glendinning, C. (2002). Comparing and contrasting the role of family carers and nurses in the domestic health care of frail older people. *Health and Social Care in the Community*, *10*(3), 144–150.

Pickard, L., King, D., & Knapp, M. (2016). The 'visibility' of unpaid care in England. *Journal of Social Work*, *16*(3), 263–282.

Powell, A., Francis-Devine, B., Foster, D., Thurley, D., Roberts, N., Loft, P., Harker, R., Mcinnes, R., Danechi, S., Kennedy, S., & Powell, T. (2020). *Informal carers* (pp. 1–45). Briefing paper 07756. https://commonslibrary.parliament.uk/research-briefings/cbp-7756/

Price, L., & Walker, L. (2015). *Chronic illness, vulnerability and social work, autoimmunity and the contemporary disease experiences*. Routledge.

Prince, M. J., Knapp, M., Guerchet, M., McCrone, P., Prina, M., Cormas-Herrera, A., Wittenberg, R., Adelaja, B., Hu, B., King, D., Rehill, A., & Salimkumar, D. (2014). *Dementia UK: Update*. Alzheimer's Society.

Public Health England. (2021). *Caring as a social determinant of health findings - From a rapid review of reviews and analysis of the GP Patient Survey*. Public Health England.

Pysklywec, A., Plante, M., Auger, C., Mortenson, W. B., Eales, J., Routhier, F., & Demers, L. (2020). The positive effects of caring for family carers of older adults: A scoping review. *International Journal of Care and Caring*, *4*(3), 349–375.

Quinn, C., Toms, G., Rippon, I., Nelis, S. M., Henderson, C., Morris, R. G., Rusted, J. M., Thom, J. M., van den Heuvel, E., Victor, C., & Clare, L. (2022). Positive experiences in dementia care-giving: Findings from the IDEAL programme. *Ageing and Society*, 1–21.

Rand, S., Zhang, W., Collins, G., Silarova, B., & Milne, A. (2022). Applying a dyadic outcomes approach to supporting older carers and care-recipients: A qualitative study of social care professionals in England. *Health and Social Care in the Community*, *30*(6), e5001–e5009.

Rapaport, J., & Manthorpe, J. (2008). Family matters: Developments concerning the role of the nearest relative and social worker under mental health law in England and Wales. *The British Journal of Social Work*, *38*(6), 1115–1131.

Rawls, J. (1999). *A theory of justice*. Oxford University Press.

Ray, M., Bernard, M., & Phillips, J. (2009). *Critical issues in social work with older people*. Palgrave Macmillan.

Ray, M., Milne, A., Beech, C., Phillips, J. E., Richards, S., Sullivan, M. P., Tanner, D., & Lloyd, L. (2015). Gerontological social work: Reflections on its role, purpose and value. *The British Journal of Social Work*, *45*(4), 1296–1312.

Ridley, J., Hunter, S., & Rosengard, A. (2010). Partners in care?: Views and experiences of carers from a cohort study of the early implementation of the Mental Health (Care and Treatment) (Scotland) Act 2003. *Health and Social Care in the Community*, *18*(5), 474–482.

Robinson, F. (2015). Care ethics, political theory, and the future of feminism. In D. Engster & M. Hammington (Eds.), *Care ethics and political theory* (pp. 293–311). Oxford University Press.

Rummery, K., & Fine, M. (2012). Care: A critical review of theory, policy and practice. *Social Policy and Administration*, *46*(3), 321–343.

Sadler, E., & McKevitt, C. (2013). 'Expert carers': An emergent normative model of the caregiver. *Social Theory & Health*, *11*(1), 40–58.

Santulli, R. B., & Blandin, K. (2015). *The emotional journey of the Alzheimer's family*. Dartmouth College.

Scourfield, P. (2005). Understanding why carers' assessments do not always take place. *Practice*, *17*(1), 15–28.

Seedat, S., & Rondon, M. (2021). Women's well-being and the burden of unpaid work. *BMJ Open*, *374*(1972).

Senior, S., Caan, W., & Gamsu, M. (2020). Welfare and well-being: Towards mental health-promoting welfare systems. *The British Journal of Psychiatry*, *216*(1), 4–5.

Sevenhuijsen, S. (1998). *Citizenship and the ethics of care: Feminist considerations on justice, morality and politics*. Routledge.

Shakespeare, T., Zeilig, H., & Mittler, P. (2019). Rights in mind: Thinking differently about dementia and disability. *Dementia*, *18*(3), 1075–1088.

Sharma, N., Chakrabarti, S., & Grover, S. (2016). Gender differences in caregiving among family - caregivers of people with mental illnesses. *World Journal of Psychiatry*, *6*(1), 7–17.

Shooshtari, S., Duncan, K. A., Roger, K., Fast, J., & Jing, H. (2017). Care-related out-of-pocket spending and caregiving consequences: Results from a Canadian population-based study. *Journal of Family and Economic Issues*, *38*(3), 405–420.

Skaff, M. M., & Pearlin, L. I. (1992). Caregiving: Role engulfment and the loss of self. *The Gerontologist*, *32*(5), 656–664.

Spencer, D., Funk, L. M., Herron, R. V., Gerbrandt, E., & Dansereau, L. (2019). Fear, defensive strategies and caring for cognitively impaired family members. *Journal of Gerontological Social Work*, 62(1), 67–85.

Stacey, C. (2005). Finding dignity in dirty work: The constraints and rewards of low-wage home care labour. *Sociology of Health & Illness*, 27(6), 831–854.

Stajduhar, K. (2011). Family carers and social difference. In D. Oliviere, B. Monroe, & S. Payne (Eds.), *Death, dying, and social differences* (2nd ed., pp. 183–190). Oxford University Press.

Starr, M., & Szebehely, M. (2017). Working longer, caring harder – The impact of 'ageing-in-place' policies on working carers in the UK and Sweden. *International Journal of Care and Caring*, 1(1), 115–119.

Stensöta, H. O. (2020). Democratic care 'for all' and trade-offs: The public solution, civil society and the market. *International Journal of Care and Caring*, 4(1), 75–89.

Stryker, S., & Burke, P. J. (2000). The past, present, and future of an identity theory. *Social Psychology Quarterly*, 63(4), 284–297.

Swanson, K. M. (1993). Nursing as informed caring for the well-being of others. *The Journal of Nursing Scholarship*, 25(4), 352–357.

Tajfel, H., & Turner, J. C. (1979). An integrative theory of inter-group conflict. In W. G. Austin & S. Worchel (Eds.), *The social psychology of inter-group relations* (pp. 33–47). Brooks/Cole.

Talic, S., Shah, S., Wild, H., Gasevic, D., Maharaj, A., Ademi, Z., Li, X., Xu, W., Mesa-Eguiagaray, I., Rostron, J.,

Theodoratou, E., Zhang, X., Motee, A., Liew, D., & Ilic, D. (2021). Effectiveness of public health measures in reducing the incidence of Covid-19, SARS-CoV-2 transmission, and Covid-19 mortality: Systematic review and meta-analysis. *BMJ*, *375*. https://doi.org/10.1136/bmj-2021-068302

Tanner, D. (2001). Sustaining the self in later life: Supporting older people in the community. *Ageing and Society*, *21*(3), 255–278.

Tanner, D. (2010). *Managing the ageing experience: Learning from older people*. Policy Press.

Tanner, D. (2013). Identity, selfhood and dementia: Messages for social work. *European Journal of Social Work*, *16*(2), 155–170.

Tanner, D. (2016). Sustaining the self in the 'fourth age': A case study. *Quality in Ageing and Older People*, *17*(3), 157–167.

Tanner, D., Ray, M., & Ward, L. (2022). 'When it comes to carers, you've got to be grateful that you've got a carer coming': Older people's narratives of self-funding social care in England. *Ageing and Society*, 1–22.

Teahan, Á., Walsh, S., Doherty, E., & O'Shea, E. (2021). Supporting family carers of people with dementia: A discrete choice experiment of public preferences. *Social Science and Medicine*, *287*. https://doi.org/10.1016/j.socscimed.2021.114359

The Health Social Care Information Centre. (2010). *Health and social care annual report and accounts*. https://www.gov.uk/government/publications/the-health-and-social-care-information-centre-annual-report-and-accounts-2009-to-2010

Thomas, C. (2007). *Sociologies of disability and illness: Contested ideas in disability studies and medical sociology.* Palgrave Macmillan.

Tronto, J. (1993). *Moral boundaries: A political argument for an ethic of care.* Routledge.

Tronto, J. (2002). The 'nanny' question in feminism. *Hypatia*, *17*(2), 34–51.

Tronto, J. (2013). *Caring democracy: Markets, equality and justice.* University Press.

Tronto, J. (2017). There is an alternative: Homines curans and the limits of neo-liberalism. *International Journal of Care and Caring*, *1*(1), 27–43.

Turner, B. S. (Ed.). (1993). *Citizenship and social theory.* Sage Publishing.

Turner, N., Schneider, J., Pollock, K., Travers, C., Perry-Young, L., & Wilkinson, S. (2020). 'Going the extra mile' for older people with dementia: Exploring the voluntary labour of homecare workers. *Dementia*, *19*(7), 2220–2233.

Twigg, J. (1993). Integrating carers into the service system: Six strategic responses. *Ageing and Society*, *13*(2), 141–170.

Twigg, J. (2000). *Bathing: The body and community care.* Routledge.

Twigg, J. (2006). *The body in health and social care.* Macmillan International Higher Education.

Twigg, J., & Atkin, K. (1994). *Carers perceived: Policy and practice in informal care.* Open University Press.

Urban, P., & Ward, L. (2020). *Care ethics, democratic citizenship and the state.* Palgrave Macmillan.

Vassilev, I., Rogers, A., Blickem, C., Brooks, H., Kapadia, D., Kennedy, A., Sanders, C., Kirk, S., & Reeves, D. (2013). Social networks, the 'work' and work force of chronic illness self-management: A survey analysis of personal communities. *PLoS One, 8*(4). https://doi.org/10.1371/journal.pone. 0059723

Ward, L., Ray, M., & Tanner, D. (2020). *The impact of self-funding on unpaid carers: Lightening the load or adding to it? Older People: Care and Self-Funding Experiences.* Briefing Paper. Brighton, University of Brighton. https://www.olderpeopleself fundingcare.com/publications/impact-of-self-funding-on-un paid-carers/

White, C. (2013). Census Analysis: Unpaid care in England and Wales, 2011 and comparison with 2001. http://www.ons.gov.uk/ peoplepopulationandcommunity/healthandsocialcare/healthcare system/articles/2011censusanalysisunpaidcareinenglandandwale s2011andcomparisonwith2001/2013-02

Whitley, E., Reeve, K., & Benzeval, M. (2021). Tracking the mental health of home-carers during the first COVID national lockdown: Evidence from a nationally representative UK survey. *Psychological Medicine,* 1–10.

Whittaker, A., & Gallagher, S. (2019). Caregiving alters immunity and stress hormones: A review of recent research. *Current Opinion in Behavioral Sciences, 28,* 93–97.

Williams, F. (2001). In and beyond new labour: Towards a new political ethics of care. *Critical Social Policy, 21*(4), 467–493.

Williams, F. (2004). *Rethinking families.* Calouste Gulbenkian Foundation.

Williams, F. (2012). Care relations and public policy: Social justice claims and social investment frames. *Families, Relationships and Societies, 1*(1), 103–119.

Williams, F. (2018). Care: Intersections of scales, inequalities and crises. *Current Sociology*, 66(4), 547–561.

Williams, A., & Bank, J. (2022). Support for working carers across the globe: The development of international standardised guidelines for the workplace. *International Journal of Care and Caring*, 6(3), 1–6.

Willis, P., & Lloyd, L. (2021). *Online advice to carers: An updated review of local authority websites in England*. School for Social Care Research, NIHR.

Willis, P., Ward, N., & Fish, J. (2011). Searching for LGBT carers: Mapping a research agenda in social work and social care. *British Journal of Social Work*, 41(7), 1304–1320.

Wilson, H. (1989). Family caregiving for a relative with Alzheimer's dementia: Coping with negative choices. *Nursing Research*, 38(2), 94–98.

Wilson, S., Marvell, R., Cox, A., & Teeman, D. (2018). *Evaluation of the Carers in Employment (CiE) project* (p. 45). https://www.scie.org.uk/carers/employment

Wittenberg, R., Knapp, M., Hu, B., Comas-Herrera, A., King, D., Rehill, A., Shi, C., Banerjee, S., Patel, A., Jagger, C., & Kingston, A. (2019). The costs of dementia in England. *International Journal of Geriatric Psychiatry*, 34(7), 1095–1103.

Xu, J., Liu, P.-J., & Beach, S. (2021). Multiple caregivers, many minds: Family discord and caregiver outcomes. *The Gerontologist*, 61(5), 661–669.

Yeandle, S., Chou, Y.-C., Fine, M., Larkin, M., & Milne, A. (2017). Editorial, care and caring: Interdisciplinary perspectives on a societal issue of global significance. *International Journal of Care and Caring*, 1(1), 3–25.

INDEX